The
Digital Detox

Reclaiming Focus and Freedom in a Hyperconnected World

By
Alaric Vadeboncoeur

The
Digital Detox

Reclaiming Focus and Freedom in a Hyperconnected World

Table of Contents

Introduction

In today's hyper-connected world, it's easy to feel like we're perpetually engulfed in a whirlwind of digital stimuli. Every day, we are bombarded by endless notifications, updates, and alerts that compete for our attention. As we stand in the midst of this digital deluge, it's crucial to pause and ask ourselves: Are we using technology, or is it using us? This book aims to explore the dynamics of digital engagement and guide you towards a more intentional and balanced relationship with technology.

The reward for immersing ourselves in this exploration is profound. Not only does it offer the potential to reclaim our time, but it also promises a more fulfilling and less cluttered mental space. Through understanding our digital habits, we can discover paths to increased focus, genuine connection, and ultimately, a more peaceful state of mind. It's time to reassess the way digital tools shape our lives and to cultivate habits that serve our true needs and aspirations.

Our modern lifestyle, intertwined with technologies, brings an unparalleled level of convenience and access—two integral aspects that define today's digital experience. Yet, ironically, this connectivity often leaves us feeling more isolated, frazzled, and distracted than ever. These paradoxes demand thoughtful examination and purposeful action. The intent is not to vilify technology but to understand it, harness it, and use it to enhance, not diminish, our human experience.

This book is not a manifesto against technological advancement. Instead, it is an invitation to pause and reflect. Why do we reach for our phones in every idle moment? How has our perception of satisfaction and contentment been molded by likes, shares, and retweets? By addressing such questions, we can start to unravel the complex relationship we have with digital devices.

Everyone's journey with technology is unique. While some may find solace in radical changes, others might only need a few mindful tweaks to witness significant improvements in their quality of life. Throughout this book, you'll encounter strategies and insights that cater to diverse needs and perspectives. From small steps like modifying notification settings to larger commitments such as digital detox retreats, the possibilities are as varied as they are impactful.

In examining the signs of digital overwhelm, we will delve into the intricacies of how technology impacts our mental health, productivity, and overall well-being. We will dissect the science behind distraction, observe the profound effects on our mental state, and explore the principles of digital minimalism. This exploration serves as the foundation for developing lasting, healthy attitudes towards technology.

Empathy and understanding are central themes as we navigate this complex landscape together. Readers who feel lost in a sea of open tabs and infinite scrolling occur will find camaraderie here. Those looking to forge a path towards digital wellness can rest assured that they're not alone. This conversation is timely, pertinent, and essential for everyone who seeks balance in a world where there's always more to consume.

The road ahead in this book will not shy away from the challenges posed by tech companies or the pervasive influence of social media. Nor will it ignore the critical roles of digital resilience and mindful engagement. Together, we will learn to set boundaries and build sustainable habits, equipping ourselves with tools to thrive without the constant beckoning of digital diversions.

By fostering a culture of mindful technology use, we embrace the opportunity for personal growth and collective well-being. The skills, techniques, and knowledge shared within these pages are not just for surviving the digital age, but for flourishing within it. Consider this your guide to cultivating a healthier, more purposeful relationship with the digital world.

This book is about reclaiming what's most valuable: our time, our connections, and our ability to live intentionally. With intention and awareness, we can choose how and when technology enriches our lives and when it must take a backseat to more pressing human experiences. Let's embark on this journey together to shed light on the path towards digital serenity and presence amidst a cacophony of technological stimuli.

Chapter 1:
The Age of Digital Overload

In an era where smartphones seem to be glued to our palms and notifications relentlessly ping for our attention, digital overload has become the new normal. We live in a seemingly interconnected world, yet many of us feel disconnected from ourselves and the moment at hand. This constant bombardment from screens has redefined how we interact, work, and even think, pushing us ever closer to a tipping point of psychological and emotional burnout. It's no wonder that many people find themselves yearning for a reprieve, craving the serenity they once found in uninterrupted human experiences. Amidst this chaos, acknowledging the pervasive nature of digital demands is the first step toward reclaiming control. By understanding the roots of this digital overwhelm, we set the stage for a deeper exploration of its impacts and the profound benefits that a more intentional relationship with technology can offer. Now is the time to pause, to breathe, and to remind ourselves that we possess the power to shape a more peaceful coexistence with the screens that dominate our lives.

Understanding Digital Overwhelm

In this age of continuous connectivity, it's easy to sometimes feel like we're drowning in a sea of digital noise. Devices beep, buzz, and blink, demanding our attention at every moment. The constant barrage can slowly edge into our lives, making it challenging to find moments of peace. But what exactly is digital overwhelm, and why does it seem to affect so many of us?

Digital overwhelm is more than just a feeling—it's a complex phenomenon impacting the mind and body. It's the sensory overload from the multitude of digital notifications, content streams, and communication channels that we've allowed into our personal spaces. Our brains, wired for survival in a world very different from today, struggle to keep up with this relentless pace. The scarcity of downtime to process this influx leads to anxiety, stress, and a sense of fragmentation in our thoughts and emotions.

Imagine a scenario where every device in your home is left running at full capacity, 24/7. The lights flicker, appliances heat up, and before long, circuits would overload, causing total shutdowns. This is a fitting metaphor for our minds in the face of digital overwhelm. Continuous stimuli leave no room for mental recharge or engagement in deep, meaningful activities, leading to consistently high stress levels and potential burnout.

Our culture seems to value constant engagement with technology as an indicator of productivity and success. It may feel that if we're not updating, browsing, liking, or responding, we're somehow falling behind. This mindset exacerbates the unending cycle of digital consumption. Yet, this constant connectivity is an illusion of productivity; the reality is different. We find ourselves distracted, less focused, and unable to maintain sustained attention on any one task.

Understanding the roots of digital overwhelm involves acknowledging how much of our lives are intertwined with screens. From remote work meetings and social media catch-ups to streaming shows and news alerts, digital interfaces dominate large portions of our daily routines. It's not just about the time spent online but also the repetitive, non-stop nature of that interaction.

Consider the myriad notifications we receive each day. With every beep or vibration, our brains release a small amount of dopamine, a neurotransmitter associated with pleasure and reward. It creates a feedback loop that tempts us to check our devices more frequently. This constant stimulation changes our brain's wiring over time, making us crave the very interruptions that cause us stress.

Moreover, digital overwhelm isn't only about the individual. It permeates relationships and workplaces too. It transforms how we interact with those around us, sometimes substituting real human connections with superficial digital interactions. At work, the omnipresence of emails and messages demands immediate attention, eroding the ability to focus deeply.

The fear of missing out (FOMO) adds another layer to this experience. It's this anxiety that something exciting or important is happening online without us, prompting us to check our devices repeatedly. Underneath this anxiety is often a broader existential question: Are we measuring our lives by real-world experiences or digital engagements?

We must remember that 'busy' and 'productive' are not synonyms. The culture of busyness fueled by digital distraction frequently leaves little room for self-reflection and genuine fulfillment. To combat digital overwhelm, it's necessary to question our relationship with technology. This involves setting intentional timeouts and creating spaces where digital devices are not the centerpiece, allowing us to reconnect with the simple, tangible aspects of life.

While technology is an incredible tool for progress, if left unchecked, it can consume our focus and peace. Recognizing digital overwhelm is the first step toward regaining balanced control over tech usage. The journey involves embracing moments of quietude, nurturing mindfulness, and fostering environments where technology serves us rather than commands us.

Ultimately, understanding digital overwhelm is about taking a step back to see the larger picture. It means recognizing the power we possess to curate a digital presence that enriches rather than depletes. Let us start by placing value on meaningful pauses and intentional engagement, leading to a more harmonious existence with technology. Through this understanding, we can begin the path to a saner, more centered digital life.

Recognizing the Signs of Digital Fatigue

In today's fast-paced, hyper-connected world, many find themselves feeling drained, overwhelmed, and even trapped by the very technologies designed to simplify our lives. Digital fatigue has become a silent epidemic, an insidious condition that creeps into the crevices of our daily existence. Identifying its signs is the first step toward reclaiming control over our tech interactions and, ultimately, our well-being.

Digital fatigue doesn't announce itself with a grand flare, but rather, it seeps in quietly, manifesting in subtle ways. One of the most common signs includes a persistent sense of mental exhaustion, even after short periods of screen time. If you find yourself feeling tired, sluggish, or unmotivated after browsing your phone or computer, you're not alone. This mental weariness often stems from the constant stimuli digital devices present.

Another indicator of digital fatigue is the struggle with concentration. It's not uncommon to start watching a video or reading an article only to realize your mind has wandered off after just a few minutes. The plethora of digital distractions out there makes sustaining focus increasingly challenging. When our brains become accustomed to rapidly shifting between tasks, the ability to concentrate takes a hit.

Physical symptoms shouldn't be overlooked either. Eyestrain, headaches, and disrupted sleep cycles are telltale signs of overexposure to screens. The blue light emitted by devices tricks our brains into thinking it's still daylight, messing with our body's natural rhythms and making restful sleep elusive. If you're waking up feeling unrested or find it hard to fall asleep, your nighttime device usage might be playing a role.

Beyond the physical and cognitive impacts lies the emotional toll of digital fatigue. Anxiety and irritability can escalate when the mind can't seem to find a moment of peace amidst the constant buzz of notifications and alerts. This relentless connectivity might also breed a sense of isolation or disconnection, paradoxically as it disconnects us from our immediate surroundings and the people present in our lives.

Further compounding this issue is the understated pressure of digital comparison. Social media platforms, while keeping us connected, also offer a curated glimpse into others' lives. The constant comparison can lead to feelings of inadequacy, heightening emotional fatigue. If you find yourself scrolling through feeds and feeling inferior or anxious about your own life, it's a definite sign that digital fatigue is setting in.

Our productivity is not immune to the effects of digital fatigue either. The illusion of multitasking—handling several digital interactions at once—can lead to decreased efficiency and increased errors. Instead of getting more done, constant task-switching wears down our cognitive resources, leaving us feeling more stressed than productive.

It's crucial to acknowledge the social dimensions of digital fatigue. As our lives become more intertwined with technology, the line between work and personal time often blurs, increasing stress levels and straining relationships. If you're finding it challenging to disconnect, or feel tied to your devices even during personal time, it's an indicator of digital fatigue infiltrating your social life.

Ultimately, recognizing these signs is about cultivating awareness. It's about pausing to reflect on how technology is affecting not just your productivity, but your mental health, relationships, and overall quality of life. By actively identifying these signals, we create a pathway to a healthier, more balanced interaction with technology.

The journey begins with self-compassion. Recognizing that digital fatigue isn't a personal failing but a common response in a tech-saturated world is empowering. From this place of understanding, we can chart a course toward more intentional tech use. This involves setting boundaries, practicing digital mindfulness, and rediscovering what it means to be truly present in our physical surroundings.

By learning to spot the signs of digital fatigue, we can begin to implement strategies that combat its effects. Prioritizing downtime, engaging in tech-free activities, and establishing periods of deliberate disconnection can all contribute to alleviating the symptoms. It's about finding a rhythm that allows for both the benefits of technology and the necessary space to breathe.

As we weave our way through this digital age, acknowledging the existence and impact of digital fatigue is crucial. It's the spark that ignites change, paving the way for a life where technology serves us— not the other way around. In recognizing these signs, you now hold the key to unlocking a future where digital well-being isn't just an aspiration but a reality.

Chapter 2:
The Impact on Mental Health

In today's digital age, the impact of technology on mental health is profound and sometimes daunting. As screens become ever-present in our lives, anxiety and depression are on the rise, largely fueled by constant connectivity and an overabundance of information. This relentless barrage can leave us feeling mentally drained and emotionally detached, making it crucial to understand how these digital interactions affect our well-being. It's not just about the sheer volume of screen time; it's the nature of engagement and the psychological effects of digital consumption that truly matter. The good news is, by adopting mindful practices, individuals can counteract these effects, finding solace and clarity in intentional digital use. Harnessing the power of technology with thoughtfulness can transform these mental health challenges into opportunities for growth and resilience, guiding us toward a more balanced and fulfilling relationship with the digital world.

Technology and Anxiety

In an age where our lives are intertwined with technology, it's no wonder that anxiety has found fertile ground to thrive. Everywhere we turn, screens demand our attention with an urgency that can be overwhelming. The constant barrage of notifications and information keeps our minds in a state of perpetual readiness, making it difficult to unwind and find peace. Technology, in its promise of connectivity and efficiency, often conversely incubates stress and worry.

Consider this: every day, people juggle multiple gadgets and platforms, from smartphones buzzing with alerts to laptops pinging with new emails. All these devices are meant to streamline our lives, yet they've created a cacophony of digital noise that many feel powerless against. This digital deluge gives rise to a unique breed of anxiety, one that is less about facing immediate threats and more about the chronic unease rooted in the "always-on" lifestyle.

How did technology, originally designed to be our ally, become a catalyst for anxiety? It's worth tracing back to the fundamental mismatch between our evolutionary wiring and modern digital innovations. Our ancestors relied on acute, short bursts of stress to survive predators. Today, instead of predators, we face an unending series of pings—a modern-day equivalent that keeps our amygdala, the brain's fear center, on high alert.

The irony lies in how technology was supposed to make life more convenient. Yet, it often feels like a relentless taskmaster, setting expectations for immediate communication and instant problem-solving. This pressure to respond promptly creates a digital version of vigilance, akin to always being on watch for danger.

Imagine, for a moment, the lingering guilt after ignoring a work email or a friend's text message. That unsettled feeling of letting someone down because we didn't immediately reciprocate. The guilt, the anxiety—it's not just paranoia; it's a pervasive, shared experience that many of us can't escape.

Moreover, the curated realities on social media contribute significantly to our anxiety. We see perfect lives and compare them with our own chaotic world, creating a warped sense of inadequacy. In this landscape, it's easy to forget the orchestrated nature of these online personas. The uplifting stories sidelined by the highlight reels exacerbate feelings of loneliness and anxiety.

On the bright side, understanding the link between technology and anxiety empowers us to take control. Knowing that our devices are designed to capture and hold our attention allows us to reclaim our focus and set boundaries. We don't need to be at the mercy of every ping or buzz.

One profound but simple strategy is adopting mindful technology use. Being conscious of how, why, and when we use our screens can dramatically shift our experience. It's about creating intentional gaps in our tech interactions, allowing time for real-life connections and activities that bring genuine joy.

Another vital aspect lies in setting personal boundaries with technology. Whether it's designating screen-free zones or committing to device-free times, these small steps cultivate a breath of fresh air in our digital-cluttered lives. It opens room for offline connections, creativity, and rest—things that reduce anxiety and build resilience against digital pressures.

Technology itself isn't inherently the culprit. Instead, it is the way we interact with it that decides its impact on our mental health. By restructuring our engagement with technology, we can transform it from an anxiety-inducing factor into a tool for productivity and peace.

Each transformative step helps counter the cycle of reactivity that technology perpetuates. As we become more deliberate about our digital consumption, we can alleviate the grip of technology-induced anxiety and foster a more balanced and fulfilling relationship with the digital world.

The journey toward a more mindful digital existence is not one that demands perfection overnight. It asks for small, sustained changes that lead to a deeper sense of peace and control over one's life. Armed with awareness and a willingness to act, individuals can indeed rewrite their narratives in this digital age, ensuring that technology serves their needs, rather than dictating their lives.

The Link Between Screen Time and Depression

It's no secret that we live in a world deeply intertwined with screens. They're in our pockets, on our desks, and sometimes even in our hands during meals. With this ubiquitous presence, a pressing question arises: how does screen time affect our mental health, particularly concerning depression? Let's explore the connection, acknowledging each layer of complexity that technology brings to our emotions.

First, consider how easy it is to get lost in the digital maze. Notifications, social media feeds, and endless streams of information can make anyone feel trapped. For many, this isn't just a harmless way to pass the time. It's a cycle that feeds a digital dependency, slowly chipping away at emotional health. Research shows that extensive screen time can correlate with increased feelings of loneliness and isolation, leading to depressive symptoms.

Our mental well-being often depends on meaningful connections and face-to-face interactions. Yet, as we spend more time interacting with our devices, these real-world interactions decrease. The irony here is palpable: in our quest for connection through social platforms, we may end up feeling more disconnected. This digital paradox leaves many individuals struggling silently, as their screens reflect only superficial connections rather than the depth they yearn for.

The content we consume plays a crucial role, too. Endless scrolling through highlight reels of others' lives can trigger unhealthy comparisons and self-doubt. "Why doesn't my life look like this?"— it's a question many ask themselves, unknowingly planting seeds of dissatisfaction and sadness. Such comparisons can skew our self-perception, making our achievements seem less meaningful.

Moreover, the pressure to be constantly available online contributes to stress levels. The expectation to respond instantly to every message and the desire to keep up with the rapid flux of digital updates can be exhausting. In this hurried state, there's little room left for self-reflection or genuine rest. Instead, individuals enter a loop of anxiety and, in severe cases, depression.

Time is another element that screens can steal away, and with it, experiences that nurture mental wellness. Imagine the peace a simple walk in nature can bring, or the sense of achievement from completing a creative project. These are routinely sacrificed at the altar of screen time. Over time, this continuous choice—even when made unconsciously—can erode our inner joy and emotional fulfillment.

Yet, screens aren't entirely to blame. Often, it's how we use them that matters most. Technology is a tool, neutral at its core. It's our mindful—or mindless—engagement with them that defines their impact. To cultivate a healthier relationship with our devices, awareness is key. Acknowledging how our screen habits make us feel is a powerful first step toward change.

Moving forward, imagine dedicating specific hours for screen-free activities. Picture reengaging with hobbies neglected in favor of screen time or scheduling regular digital detox days. These small adjustments can gradually restore balance, offering a reprieve to nourish our minds and souls.

Balancing screen time in our digitized world is challenging but possible. It involves making conscious choices to prioritize well-being over convenience. This journey may require experimenting with different strategies, self-assessing regularly, and even seeking support from others on the same path toward lessening screen-induced blues.

Chapter 3:
Productivity in a Connected World

In our hyper-connected era, the quest for productivity has become both a challenge and an opportunity. As we navigate through endless notifications and digital distractions, it's tempting to believe the myth of multitasking—that somehow handling multiple tasks simultaneously equals efficiency. Yet, genuine productivity requires a more mindful approach. By embracing a single-task focus, we begin to reclaim our attention in a world that constantly demands it. It's not about shunning technology but about leveraging it thoughtfully to foster deeper concentration and a sense of fulfillment. When we integrate mindful practices into our digital interactions, we carve out spaces for creativity and clarity amid the noise. This intentional shift doesn't just boost our output; it fundamentally transforms our relationship with technology, empowering us to navigate our virtual worlds with purpose and peace.

Multitasking Myths

In our hyperconnected world, the concept of multitasking has become almost mythical. We glorify it as an essential skill required to thrive amid the relentless barrage of emails, notifications, and updates. Yet, embracing multitasking as a productivity tool is one of the most persistent misconceptions of modern life. Far from making us more efficient, multitasking can undermine our ability to work effectively and creatively.

When we try to juggle multiple tasks, what we're actually doing is rapidly switching our focus from one task to another. This switch comes at a cost. Cognitive psychologists have shown that task-switching can lead to significant decreases in productivity, often referred to as "switching costs." Each shift in focus takes time and mental energy, derivatives of attention being wasted in the transition. Such patterns not only drain personal resources but also diminish the quality of our output.

Moreover, multitasking can impair cognitive ability more than being high on marijuana, according to some studies. The human brain is not designed to perform multiple complex processes simultaneously. It can severely impact our short-term memory, impede our learning, and erode our ability to think deeply and creatively. Instead of stretching our intellectual capacity, what we often achieve is a diluted attention span.

But where does this myth originate? It may stem from a cultural narrative that equates busyness with significance. In a society obsessed with doing, slowing down feels risky, even lazy. The always-on nature of modern work culture valorizes the constant bustle, rewarding those who can seemingly handle 10 things at once. Yet, this busyness does not equate to real productivity.

Interestingly, the misunderstanding extends even into our understanding of how our own technology works. Despite advances in tech that have streamlined many aspects of our professional and personal lives, the psychological cost of managing multiple digital interactions remains high. Notifications pinging from our phones, emails stacking up with subject lines screaming for our attention — they are the perfect storm for disjointed focus.

Let's dissect an important difference: real multitasking, such as walking while listening to music, versus pseudo-multitasking, such as writing a report while continuously checking emails. The former pairs complementary activities that can co-exist because they don't compete for the same cognitive resources. The latter, however, involves activities that vie for the brain's limited attention, leading to reduced efficiency in both tasks.

So, what do we do with this information? After all, responsibilities won't desist, and our devices aren't going anywhere. The first step to overcoming the myth of multitasking is to embrace single-tasking. Focus deeply on one thing at a time, diving completely into it and allowing your mind to engage fully. Be present and intentional in your actions.

Single-tasking is daunting in an era that feels like a blur. However, its power lies in simplifying our mental load, resulting in a more profound engagement with our work. It allows us to complete tasks more quickly and with higher quality, improving our overall sense of accomplishment and fulfillment.

A strategy to bolster single-tasking involves setting specific times for checking emails and responding to messages. Delineate clear boundaries by allocating dedicated focus periods that are devoid of interruptions, creating an environment where deep work can flourish. Such discipline in your workflow isn't just about controlling technology; it's about reclaiming some semblance of clarity in a digital maze.

Additionally, cultivating a habit of reflection can help resist the lure of multitasking. Take a step back to identify times when you have fallen into multitasking traps. Analyze these moments, understanding both the triggers and the impacts. This awareness can be empowering, giving you the tools to break free from multitasking tendencies.

It's essential to recognize that this isn't about rejecting efficiency or contemporary ways of working but rather about redefining efficiency on more human terms. We shouldn't feel guilty for slowing down, nor embarrassed to admit that our limits have been reached. Instead, we can view this acknowledgment as a path to better well-being and enriched productivity.

In this connected world, where the pressure to multitask is ever-present, dispelling these myths is an act of self-care and resilience. By rejecting the illusion of multitasking, we open doors to more focused, deliberate, and meaningful engagement with our tasks. More importantly, it allows us to reclaim our most valuable asset: our attention.

Reclaiming Focus with Mindfulness

In a world where digital distractions attempt to hijack our attention every second, reclaiming focus through mindfulness emerges as a beacon of hope. Mindfulness isn't just a trend or another task to add to your already long to-do list—it's a way of life that invites you to live in the moment. At its core, mindfulness is about cultivating an awareness of the present, allowing us to recognize when our minds wander and gently guiding them back.

Imagine sitting in a bustling café. Your phone buzzes, a reminder, maybe a news alert, or a friend's message. It's tempting to give in and check. But mindfulness asks us to pause, notice the impulse, and decide deliberately whether to engage. In this space between stimulus and response lies the true power of choice. By consciously deciding to focus elsewhere, we train our minds to manage distractions better, building our capacity for sustained attention.

The beauty of mindfulness is its accessibility. You don't require specialized equipment or elaborate prep to start. Begin where you are, with what you have. Maybe it's a few deep breaths to center yourself before diving into a task, or perhaps it's taking a quiet moment to appreciate your surroundings during your morning coffee. Each small step contributes to a more focused and intentional life.

However, truly integrating mindfulness in our daily routine requires that we understand its importance beyond occasional moments. Our digital devices operate on an urgency culture, tricking us into believing that every notification demands immediate attention. Mindfulness teaches us otherwise. It trains us to value what's truly important, helping to sift through the noise of the digital world and concentrate on what really matters.

Mindfulness isn't just about ignoring distractions; it's about changing our relationship with them. Recognize that our minds naturally drift—that's human nature. When distractions occur, instead of chastising ourselves, we can acknowledge the wandering mind with compassion. With practice, this awareness fosters patience and reduces the anxiety of feeling constantly behind or overwhelmed.

Developing a mindfulness practice can act as a buffer against the cognitive chaos many of us experience. Research has shown that consistent mindfulness practice can restructure the brain, enhancing areas responsible for attention and emotional regulation. This neuroplasticity offers hope for those struggling to keep digital distractions at bay, proving that we're capable of change and growth even in a rapidly evolving digital landscape.

Consider starting a daily mindfulness regimen. It doesn't have to be intensive—even setting aside two to five minutes each day can make a significant impact. These moments of reprieve allow for reflection, rejuvenating your capacity for focus. Engage in mindful breathing, or perhaps try a body scan meditation to reconnect with yourself.

As you embark on this mindfulness journey, you'll likely notice subtle changes. Tasks that once seemed daunting might become more manageable. You might find it easier to tune out the relentless hum of digital chatter. Gradually, the inner silence and clarity that mindfulness fosters lead not only to increased productivity but also to a more balanced, serene life.

Incorporating mindfulness into the workplace isn't just reserved for individuals. Teams and organizations are beginning to recognize its value. Imagine a work environment where meetings start with a moment of silence, or employees are encouraged to take digital detox breaks. Such practices not only boost focus and productivity but also elevate the overall sense of well-being among team members.

But how do we begin this cultural shift toward mindfulness amid a digital frenzy? It starts by championing small changes—both individually and collectively. Prioritize necessary digital tasks and allow intentional pauses in between. Replace the habit of jumping from one screen to another with mindful transitions, taking a deep breath and resetting focus.

Embracing mindfulness positions us not in opposition to technology, but in harmony with it. It's about creating a tech-life balance that supports rather than undermines our mental and emotional health. While technology offers conveniences, it's mindfulness that nudges us towards a more considerate usage pattern, ensuring that we're still the custodians of our time and attention.

As you navigate the ever-connected world, remember: mindfulness is not about perfection, but progress. It involves recognizing patterns, understanding tendencies, and crafting a more intentional presence both online and offline. So pause, breathe, and reclaim your focus— one mindful moment at a time.

Chapter 4:
What is Digital Minimalism?

Digital minimalism is a philosophy that empowers individuals to break free from the relentless, mindless consumption of technology and recapture a more intentional, fulfilling approach to digital life. Rooted in the idea of simplifying one's digital environment, it emphasizes a values-driven use of technology, where tools and apps serve the user's deeply held purposes rather than dictate them. By adopting digital minimalism, individuals can create a life enriched with meaningful interactions and purposeful technology use, ultimately fostering a sense of tranquility and focus often drowned out by digital commotion. It's about making conscious choices that reflect personal intentions and priorities, leaving room for creativity and connection that extends beyond the digital domain. In essence, digital minimalism invites us to reclaim our time and attention, redirecting them toward endeavors that matter most. Through this mindful approach, we cultivate a more balanced relationship with technology, ensuring that it enhances rather than hinders our daily lives.

Core Principles of Digital Minimalism

Digital minimalism is more than a trend; it's a philosophy for navigating the constant barrage of digital inputs in our modern lives. At its heart, digital minimalism is about intentionality. It's about making calculated choices regarding what technology to use, and crucially, when to put it aside. For individuals feeling overwhelmed by digital noise, these core principles can be a lifeline, offering a path to greater peace and focus.

The first principle is choice. Digital minimalism encourages you to choose the technology that adds real value to your life, rather than letting technology choose you. This involves identifying your tools and platforms that truly serve your goals. For some, this could mean committing to a single form of social media that fosters meaningful connections rather than scattering efforts across several platforms. For others, it might be about selecting apps or tools that streamline productivity without siphoning too much attention from the task at hand.

Another principle is constraint. While it may seem counterintuitive, imposing limitations on our tech use can lead to greater freedom. By setting boundaries, such as designated tech-free times or spaces, we can reclaim control over our attention. For instance, creating screen-free zones in the home can foster more engaging interactions with family and friends, allowing deep conversations without the disruption of electronic notifications. Constraints can seem restrictive at first but eventually lend themselves to a lifestyle that prioritizes depth over breadth.

Mindfulness, the third core principle, ties deeply into the practice of digital minimalism. It's about engaging with technology consciously, being aware of our habits, and understanding the triggers that pull us online, often mindlessly. Practicing mindfulness can transform our relationship with technology, allowing us to interact with it more purposefully. This might mean taking a moment to breathe and consider the impact before launching an application or scrolling through a feed, thereby cultivating a more deliberate use of digital tools.

Simplification plays a critical role in digital minimalism, urging you to streamline your digital environment. By eliminating clutter, you're left with the essentials that best support your values and goals. This could involve cleaning out email inboxes, organizing digital files into intuitive systems, or unsubscribing from newsletters that no longer serve a purpose. Simplification reduces cognitive load and frees up mental space for creativity and deep work.

Intentionality also extends to the content we consume. Another principle of digital minimalism involves curating your information diet. Just as you might carefully select what you eat for your physical health, the information you choose to consume affects your mental well-being. This principle recommends being selective, opting for content that enriches your life, and being critical of the news, social media, or entertainment that may not always benefit your mental space.

The concept of solitude is pivotal in digital minimalism and often misunderstood. Solitude isn't about being lonely; it's about carving out time away from digital noise to process thoughts and emotions. It's about reflecting on experiences without interference and considering what truly matters to you. In our hyper-connected world, true solitude is a rarity, but it's essential for personal growth and well-being.

Finally, digital minimalism invites us to embrace intentional disconnection. The power of unplugging regularly, whether for a few hours or entire weekends, cannot be overstated. This principle champions the idea that disconnecting allows us to reconnect with the physical world and the people around us. It's about making space for offline pleasures and rediscovering the lost art of boredom, which can lead to creativity and personal reflection.

In essence, digital minimalism isn't about rejecting technology outright. Instead, it encourages a conscious approach to its use, reminding us to balance our digital engagements with the richness of the analog world. As you begin to embrace these principles, you'll likely uncover a newfound clarity and purpose, navigating the digital landscape with confidence and calm. Making technology work for you, rather than the other way around, ultimately fosters a more fulfilling relationship with the digital world.

The Benefits of Minimalist Tech Use

Minimalist tech use offers a gateway to freedom in a world that often feels overwhelmingly connected. As we navigate the crowded digital landscape, filled with constant notifications, endless updates, and infinite scrolls, the simplicity of using technology in a minimalist way can be profoundly liberating. It provides us with the opportunity to reclaim our time, attention, and ultimately, our lives. Moving towards digital minimalism doesn't mean rejecting technology, but rather embracing a more intentional and purposeful way of engaging with it.

One of the most compelling benefits of minimalist tech use is the enhancement of mental clarity. When we're no longer bombarded with a continuous influx of information, our minds have space to wander, to unlock creativity, and to focus deeply on activities that truly matter. Imagine starting your morning without the urge to check emails or social media. Instead, you might dedicate time to reflection or to activities that set a peaceful tone for your day. Such practices nurture mindfulness, which has been shown to significantly reduce stress and improve overall mental health.

Furthermore, adopting minimalist tech habits fosters better focus and productivity. In a world where multitasking is often glorified, the truth is that frequent context switching diminishes our ability to concentrate effectively. By stripping away unnecessary digital clutter and interruptions, we can regain our capacity for deep, uninterrupted work. This leads not only to improved output but also to greater satisfaction in the work we undertake. Tasks become more than just items to tick off our list; they transform into opportunities for absorbing engagement and accomplishment.

Minimalist tech use also supports healthier personal relationships. The omnipresence of digital devices in our social interactions often creates barriers rather than building connections. Whether it's the phone ringing during a dinner or the urge to capture every moment instead of experiencing it, technology sometimes detracts from genuine interactions. By intentionally choosing moments to disconnect, we pave the way for deeper, more meaningful relationships. We become more present, listen more intently, and engage more fully with the people around us.

Importantly, minimalist tech use is a powerful tool for reclaiming time. We often underestimate the cumulative hours spent navigating feeds and responding to notifications. With a conscious effort to minimize these habits, we find pockets of time that can be redirected towards activities that enrich our lives: hobbies, exercise, face-to-face social interactions, or even simple relaxation. The ability to choose how we spend our time, free from the dictates of digital demands, fosters a greater sense of autonomy and control over our daily existence.

In addition to personal benefits, minimalism in tech use promotes a more sustainable relationship with technology. In an era of constant upgrades and the throwaway culture surrounding gadgets, taking a minimalist approach encourages us to make more deliberate choices. By prioritizing quality and longevity over novelty, we contribute positively to reducing e-waste and championing more environmentally conscious consumption. This awareness not only benefits the planet but also aligns our tech usage with our broader values.

The practice of digital minimalism aligns closely with cultivating gratitude and intentionality in our lives. When technology is used sparingly and deliberately, it becomes a tool that serves our needs rather than dominating them. We begin to appreciate the remarkable capabilities of tech without feeling beholden to it. This shift in perspective fosters a profound sense of appreciation for both the digital world and the richness of the offline world that is often overshadowed.

Transitioning to minimalist tech use isn't about rigidly restricting our digital interactions but rather about finding balance. It's recognizing the ways in which technology enhances our lives while setting boundaries to prevent it from encroaching on our wellbeing. Digital minimalism offers a pathway to not only survive but thrive in our hyper-connected age. By embracing this mindset, we open the door to a life brimming with presence, intentionality, and peace.

Chapter 5:
The Science of Distraction

As we delve into the science of distraction, it's crucial to understand the intricate ways our devices manipulate our attention and influence our neural pathways. In an age where every ping and notification fights for a slice of our mental focus, recognizing these subtle hijackers becomes essential. Our brains, wired for novelty and instant gratification, often struggle to resist the lure of constant digital engagement. This relentless assault on our attention impairs our ability to concentrate, fragmenting our thoughts and reducing our capacity for deep work. Neural studies reveal how sustained attention is disrupted, leading to a cycle of perpetual distraction that snags us in its grip. Yet, by better grasping the neurobiological underpinnings of focus, we arm ourselves with the knowledge to reclaim our cognitive territory. Understanding this dynamic empowers us to consciously design our environments and habits, fostering a deeper, more intentional relationship with technology that enriches rather than detracts from our lives.

How Devices Hijack Our Attention

In the modern age, our attention has become one of the most sought-after commodities. With the rise of digital devices, the ability to focus has become increasingly elusive. Each ping and notification is meticulously designed to draw us in, prompting a quick look that often turns into a prolonged engagement. It's not merely the devices themselves but the sophisticated tactics employed by tech companies to capture and hold our attention that leads to this distraction.

The design of digital interfaces is not arbitrary. Instead, it's rooted in deep psychological insights whose sole aim is to capture our attention. Consider the endless scroll feature on social media, akin to pulling a lever on a slot machine. This mechanism taps into our reward system, making each scroll a potential gateway to something interesting or exciting. As a result, we find ourselves trapped in a loop, scrolling, swiping, and refreshing, often without conscious thought.

Our brains are hardwired to respond to novel stimuli. In digital environments, notifications serve as triggers that hijack our attention. They activate areas of the brain linked to curiosity and surprise, compelling us to check our devices repeatedly. This constant vigilance reshapes how we think and process information. Rather than engaging in deep, meaningful thought, we skim the surface, jumping from one thing to the next without truly absorbing any of it.

The lure of multitasking can deceive us into believing that we're being productive. We switch between apps, respond to messages, and consume news feeds, all in a matter of minutes. However, this fractured approach cripples our productivity. Studies show that the human brain is not adept at handling multiple tasks simultaneously. Instead, each switch incurs a cognitive "switching cost," eroding our ability to perform tasks effectively and diminishing our overall cognitive capacity.

Part of the problem entails how devices blend seamlessly into our daily routines. They become extensions of ourselves, omnipresent and demanding attention at all times. Notifications from critical apps mix with trivial updates, blurring the line between essential and non-essential distractions. This blending creates a constant stream of interruptions and demands, making it difficult to engage in single-focused tasks.

One might wonder why it's so difficult to resist these devices. The answer lies in the feedback loops engineered into the technology itself. Each interaction we have with our devices releases a small dose of dopamine in our brain. This "feel-good" neurotransmitter is meant to reinforce behavior, nudging us to repeat actions that lead to a dopamine release. Unfortunately, tech companies have perfected the delivery of these dopamine hits, urging us to return to our screens again and again.

Additionally, the social aspect of device usage plays a significant role in hijacking our attention. The fear of missing out (FOMO) keeps us tethered to our screens, anxious not to miss updates, messages, or opportunities. Social media platforms, in particular, capitalize on this anxiety, perpetuating a cycle where the more we engage, the more we feel the need to stay connected. This relentless pursuit of social validation leaves us mentally exhausted, yet unable to disconnect.

Devices also manipulate time perception, contributing to the hijacking of our attention. Minutes turn into hours as we become engrossed in content tailored to push our emotional buttons. Algorithms prioritize material that provokes strong reactions—content that can keep us engaged longer, whether through outrage, joy, or laughter. This emotional tug keeps us locked in a cycle of consumption, often at the expense of our time and well-being.

Yet, in understanding how devices hijack our attention, we regain power to intervene. Awareness is the first step towards change. By recognizing the deliberate mechanics at play, we can begin to reshape our relationships with our devices. Mindfulness and intentionality can become allies in this fight. By establishing clear boundaries and taking proactive steps to moderate usage, we start dismantling the control devices have over us.

Consider adopting intentional 'tech breaks,' where you consciously step away from your devices. Use this time to engage in activities that deepen focus and presence—reading a book, meditating, or simply taking a walk without your phone. These moments of disconnection can help reset your attention span, creating space for deeper thought and reflection.

Furthermore, customizing your device settings to suit your focus needs can create a buffer against constant distractions. Disable unnecessary notifications, shed unwanted apps, and create screen-free zones in your daily life. These small but strategic adjustments can foster environments conducive to concentration and tranquility.

Finally, strive to develop a technology use framework that aligns with your values and goals. Reflect on what truly matters and aim to use technology as a tool that serves you rather than dictates your time and attention. Lean into authentic connections, whether through engaging with a supportive community offline or choosing platforms that enrich instead of drain your energy.

Although devices are intricately designed to hijack our attention, this doesn't mean we're powerless against them. With mindful practices and proactive measures, we can reclaim our focus and cultivate a balanced, fulfilling relationship with technology.

The Neurobiology of Focus

In a world that constantly pulls our attention in myriad directions, understanding the neurobiology of focus is crucial. It's not just about disciplining our minds but recognizing the biological symphony that allows us to zero in on the task at hand. Modern neuroscience has shed light on what happens in the brain when we concentrate, providing insights into how we can cultivate this skill amidst digital chaos. At its core, focus is an intricate interaction between different brain regions, all harmonized to filter out distractions and make sense of the deluge of information constantly vying for our attention.

The ability to focus begins in the prefrontal cortex, the brain's CEO of sorts, which is tasked with managing attention, memory, and the organization of tasks. This frontal lobe region acts as our mental command center, determining how well we can initiate concentration and maintain it over time. However, the prefrontal cortex doesn't work in isolation. It partners with deeper structures like the thalamus, which serves as a relay station, and the reticular activating system, which regulates our state of wakefulness and alertness.

Dopamine, a neurotransmitter most commonly associated with pleasure and reward, plays a significant role in focus and attention. It operates like a feedback loop, rewarding us for staying attentive by releasing feel-good chemicals when we accomplish a task or make progress towards a goal. This biochemical reward system can, in turn, enhance motivation and attention, creating a cycle that encourages sustained focus.

However, our brains are also wired to seek novelty, which can be an evolutionary hangover from times when spotting new stimuli could mean the difference between survival and danger. This natural tendency is one reason why it's so easy for our minds to wander, especially in today's digital age where constant buzzes and pings from our devices tap directly into this primal impulse. Technology often revels in exploiting this neurological quirk, presenting us with endless new information to draw us away from our intended focus.

In a digitally infused environment, distractions are mere taps away. But it's worth noting that not all distractions are equal. Some unexpected interruptions can invigorate our cognitive processes, provided they are brief and limited in number. These kinds of interruptions might reset our attention spans, allowing us to return to a task with renewed focus. This perspective can be liberating as it allows us to recalibrate every so often and achieve deeper insight after a small cognitive break.

Furthermore, the role of emotion in focus cannot be underestimated. The limbic system, which includes the amygdala and hippocampus, links emotions with our memories and decisions. When we're emotionally invested in what we're doing, these brain regions help enhance our focus. Passion and purpose are, therefore, powerful tools in the art of concentration. When an activity resonates deeply with us, our ability to focus intensely feels less forced and more organic.

On a practical level, nurturing the neurobiological processes of focus can be transformative. Regular mindfulness practices have been shown to increase gray matter in regions of the brain associated with focus, suggesting that such exercises can bolster our natural attentional capabilities. Techniques like meditation can enhance our capacity for sustained attention and emotional regulation, equipping us with more robust mental tools to counteract the distractions posed by a tech-laden world.

Given the brain's plastic nature, our focus can be trained much like a muscle. Introducing short periods of deep work, where one deliberately focuses without interruption, strengthens the neural wiring needed for sustained attentional focus. Over time, such exercises can significantly enhance our ability not just to concentrate but to do so consistently and with less effort.

It's also essential to consider the impact of our physical state on our ability to focus. Sleep, nutrition, and exercise are foundational in maintaining cognitive sharpness. Lack of sleep, for instance, can dull the prefrontal cortex's efficiency, making it more challenging to manage distractions and maintain concentration. Similarly, regular physical activity promotes better blood circulation, essentially feeding the brain with the oxygen and nutrients necessary for optimal performance.

What emerges from understanding the neurobiology of focus is not just a compelling scientific narrative but an actionable framework. By aligning our practices with what science tells us about our brains, we become more adept at crafting environments—both internal and external—that foster calm and focus rather than chaos and distraction.

Ultimately, reclaiming our focus in the digital age is a journey back to ourselves. By tuning into the biological nuances that underline our cognitive capabilities, we can mindfully steer through the torrent of digital noise that seeks to drown out the quiet voice of our deepest intentions and desires. Armed with the knowledge of how our brains work best, we are empowered to create strategies that not only buffer us against distraction but also propel us toward a more balanced and fulfilling relationship with technology.

Chapter 6:
Setting Boundaries with Technology

In our hyper-connected world, setting boundaries with technology isn't just advisable—it's vital for nurturing mental clarity and emotional well-being. As digital devices entwine with nearly every aspect of our lives, creating deliberate constraints serves as an anchor amidst the storm of notifications and online demands. By carving out screen-free zones and embracing digital downtime, you invite moments of peace and presence that technology often neglects. Consider these boundaries as gateways to reclaiming your attention and intention. They're not rigid rules but flexible frameworks that adapt to your life's rhythm, helping you cultivate a healthier, more intentional relationship with digital tools. Embracing these changes demands courage and commitment, yet the rewards—a more focused, serene, and fulfilling existence—are well worth the effort.

Creating Screen-Free Zones

In the constant hum of our digitally connected lives, finding refuge might seem impossible. Yet, creating screen-free zones can be your sanctuary. Imagine spaces in your home where the glow of screens can't intrude—a living room filled with the warmth of conversation, a bedroom conducive to restful sleep, or a dining area where meals and memories are shared with undivided attention. The very act of establishing such zones acknowledges the need to carve out peace amidst the digital clamor.

Screen-free zones are more than mere physical spaces; they are an intentional design for a more mindful existence. By relegating technology to designated areas, you take a stand for your well-being and prioritize what truly matters. The benefits extend beyond the tangible; they offer profound psychological relief, making these spaces a retreat for the mind. It's about setting up a boundary that values presence over digital distractions.

Creating these zones requires commitment, but the payoff can be significant. Start small. Choose an area in your home where it makes the most sense. You might begin with the dining room table, a sacred place for family interactions. Encourage everyone to leave their devices at a designated spot before meals. Notice the conversations that unfold and the silence that holds room for real thought without the interruption of notifications.

These zones can also be transformative for personal time. Your bedroom, for example, should be a haven for rest and reflection, not a place where last-minute emails and social media scrolls disrupt your peace. Consider instituting a no-screen rule at least an hour before bed. Replace digital devices with books, journals, or a simple meditation practice. Observe how the quality of your sleep improves and how waking up becomes a gentler experience.

Adopting screen-free zones isn't just for homes; workplaces too can benefit. Designate certain areas of the office as tech-free to foster creativity and focus. Whether it's a lounge where colleagues brainstorm freely without digital intrusion or a corner for solo reflection, these spaces can significantly enhance productivity and mental well-being. By allowing minds to wander and discuss ideas in real-time, innovative thinking becomes more robust.

For families, screen-free zones cultivate deeper connections. It's not just about banning devices but also about inviting everyone to engage differently. Encourage outdoor play, board games, or collaborative cooking sessions. Notice how these activities enrich familial bonds and provide a kind of connection that no technology can replicate. Children, especially, benefit from these interactions as they learn to balance digital lives with meaningful, real-world experiences.

While creating screen-free zones, communication and consistency are key. Discuss the rationale with family members or colleagues and involve them in the process. Understand that it's not about demonizing technology but about choosing when and how to engage with it. Approach the transition with flexibility, allowing for adjustments as you find what works best for everyone involved.

Implementing these zones effectively also requires clear guidelines. Define what constitutes a screen and how the rules apply. Laptops, tablets, and phones are obvious, but consider the nuances of smart speakers or digital readers. Make sure everyone agrees on these terms, so there's no confusion. Reinforce the purpose: enhancing quality time and mental rejuvenation.

Over time, the reverberations of these screen-free spaces can be felt beyond immediate settings. There's a ripple effect where making conscious choices in one area compels others, fostering a culture of intentional technology use. You find yourself more mindful when re-entering digital spaces, carrying the principles of the screen-free zone with you. It's a gentle reminder that balance is within reach, and it's yours to shape.

Some might wonder if these zones lead to missing out, but the real loss comes from a life filled only by screens. By reinforcing the presence of physical spaces, we gain much more than we lose—depth in interactions, clarity of mind, and an appreciation for the world around us that can get overshadowed by constant connectivity.

Creating screen-free zones is not about abrupt digital detoxes, but a gradual shift towards more impactful engagements with both technology and each other. It's a step towards reclaiming your life from the clutch of screens, giving you the freedom to choose when technology serves you and when it supplants what matters most.

In conclusion, screen-free zones are both a refuge and an act of defiance against the overwhelming demands of the digital world. They offer pockets of calm where you can breathe, think, and be without the relentless rush of information. Let these spaces be your allies in the pursuit of a life led with intention and mindfulness. And as you cultivate them, watch how presence, peace, and personal growth follow naturally in their wake.

The Importance of Digital Downtime

Amidst the constant hum of notifications, pings, and updates, carving out digital downtime is more essential than ever. It's not simply about turning off devices—it's about reclaiming our mental landscape. Technological boundaries are crucial not just for our productivity but for preserving our mental health. We live in an era where being perpetually connected feels like a requirement, yet this connectivity often exacerbates stress and fatigue. By prioritizing digital downtime, we begin to honor our need for rest and reflection, something modern life tends to overlook.

Imagine your mind as a muscle. Constant exertion, without adequate rest, leads to fatigue and decreased performance. The same principle applies to our brains, especially as they navigate the unrelenting deluge of information through screens. Digital downtime serves as the much-needed respite, allowing cognitive functions to recover and recharge. This pause not only enhances mental clarity but also fosters creativity. It's in moments of quiet reflection that innovative ideas often surface, unobscured by the noise of digital distraction.

The concept of digital downtime encourages us to differentiate between urgent and important. In a world where everything seems urgent, it's easy to lose sight of what truly matters. By setting intentional breaks from technology, we grant ourselves the opportunity to refocus and realign with our values and priorities. This might look like a designated tech-free day each week or simple daily practices such as turning off devices during meals. The specific practices are less important than the intention behind them—to create a space where technology supports rather than controls our lives.

Moreover, digital downtime plays a pivotal role in nurturing our emotional well-being. Constant connectivity can lead to a heightened sense of anxiety and restlessness. In contrast, moments of solitude and disconnection allow us to tune into our emotions without external interference. This can lead to a more profound understanding of our feelings and a greater capacity for self-compassion. When we're perpetually engaged in digital activities, we risk numbing ourselves to deeper emotional experiences, potentially stalling personal growth.

The physiological benefits of digital downtime should not be underestimated. Studies have shown that even brief periods of disconnecting can reduce cortisol levels, the body's primary stress hormone. This physiological shift underscores the importance of integrating digital downtime into our daily lives. Over time, these practices can contribute significantly to overall health, reducing the risk of stress-related illnesses and promoting longevity.

We often underestimate the extent to which technology influences our social connections. While digital tools offer unique opportunities for communication, they can't replace the depth of face-to-face interactions. Digital downtime opens up space for authentic human connections. Whether it's having a conversation without the distraction of screens or engaging in community activities, these interactions foster a sense of belonging and strengthen social bonds. In a world that often feels disconnected despite its connectivity, nurturing these relationships is vital.

Another crucial aspect to consider is the impact of digital downtime on sleep quality. Exposure to screens, especially before bedtime, can disrupt our natural sleep rhythms due to the emission of blue light. By instituting a tech-free period before sleep, we facilitate better sleep hygiene, ensuring that our bodies and minds receive the rest they require. This simple adjustment can drastically improve our mood, cognitive functioning, and overall quality of life.

As we introduce digital downtime into our routines, it's important to cultivate a sense of patience and self-kindness. Shifting habits in a tech-dominated world is no small feat, and it's natural to encounter resistance—both from ourselves and those around us. Embracing small, consistent changes can make the process more manageable. Over time, these incremental adjustments accumulate, leading to more profound shifts in how we engage with the digital world.

In the end, the journey toward integrating digital downtime is deeply personal. What works for one person might not work for another. The key is to remain curious and open to experimentation. Perhaps it starts with turning off email notifications after work hours, followed by a commitment to tech-free family dinners. These moments of intentionality can become powerful catalysts for change, ultimately contributing to a more balanced and fulfilling relationship with technology.

The beauty of digital downtime lies in its ability to reconnect us with a quieter, more thoughtful way of being. It invites us to slow down, breathe, and inhabit our lives more fully. It is an invitation to return to presence—where we can savor simple joys, nurture our inner selves, and rediscover our place in the world. In choosing to disconnect, if only for a while, we create the space needed to reconnect with what truly matters. This is the gift of digital downtime—a chance to pause and revisit our priorities with fresh eyes and renewed purpose.

Chapter 7:
Creating a Balanced Digital Life

To create a balanced digital life, it's vital to engage in intentional technology use that aligns with our values and aspirations. In a world buzzing with digital noise, finding harmony is an individual journey where mindfulness becomes our compass. Begin by prioritizing meaningful connections; face-to-face interactions often nourish us far more profoundly than a hundred likes. Evaluate your online habits, reflecting on activities that truly enrich your life. Craft a customized digital plan that includes scheduled screen-free times, allowing space for creativity and real-world engagements. By consciously weaving technology into the fabric of our lives, we can harness its possibilities without becoming ensnared by it, achieving greater focus and emotional well-being as we stride toward a fulfilled existence.

Prioritizing Meaningful Connections

In the crowded digital world we navigate daily, prioritizing meaningful connections stands as a beacon of intentional living. So often, we find ourselves juggling an endless loop of notifications, each vying for our attention, with little thought given to the quality of these interactions. It's easy to get caught in the web of virtual communication, leaving many feeling more isolated than ever before, despite the ubiquitous connectivity. But let's shift this perspective and explore how we can foster connections that enrich our lives, rather than detracting from them.

One essential step to creating meaningful connections is shifting our focus from quantity to quality. It's not about how many friends or followers we have, but about nurturing the relationships that truly matter. Consider the people who bring joy, support, and growth to your life. Consciously allocate time to deepen these relationships, both online and offline. Sometimes, it's as simple as a heartfelt message or a phone call that brings someone closer, reminding both parties of the bond they share.

Human beings are inherently social creatures, wired for connection and interaction. Digital tools can either bridge these connections or create a barrier. The choice lies in how we use them. Instead of letting digital interfaces dictate our interactions, we can employ them thoughtfully to enhance our connections. Plan online meetups with distant loved ones, or use video calls to share meaningful life events. Technology, after all, is just a tool - it's how we wield it that defines its impact on our relationships.

Creating spaces free from digital interruption can also help build stronger connections. Imagine sharing a meal, undistracted by screens, with a friend or family member. The connection deepens through shared moments of laughter or meaningful conversation. Such intentional face-to-face interactions help us feel viewed and valued, fostering emotional connections that technology alone cannot replicate.

Moreover, it's crucial to recognize that while digital communication is convenient, it often lacks the emotional nuances of in-person interactions. A text or email can be misunderstood without the context of tone or body language. By prioritizing real-life encounters where possible, we allow for richer communication and stronger relationships. When in-person meetings aren't feasible, taking a moment to craft thoughtful and considerate messages can bridge the gap, ensuring that the essence of our intent is preserved.

Joining communities with shared interests also plays a significant role in cultivating meaningful connections. These communities, whether physical or digital, offer a space where individuals can connect over a common goal or passion. It's in these spaces that one finds camaraderie and support, a reminder that they aren't alone in their journey. The exchange of ideas and experiences within these groups often leads to profound and lasting relationships.

Yet, it's crucial to acknowledge the role of authenticity in meaningful connections. The digital realm often tempts us to present idealized versions of ourselves. However, genuine connections thrive on transparency and vulnerability. Being open about our struggles and triumphs invites others to do the same, creating a foundation of trust and understanding. It's liberating to engage with others when masks are dropped and real stories are shared, paving the way for truly meaningful interactions.

Reflecting on our own social habits can illuminate where adjustments are needed. Are there people we used to stay connected with who bring happiness or fulfillment? Or others who may drain our energy? Regular reflection allows us to recalibrate our social investments, nurturing connections that align with our values and interests. This deliberate curation not only balances our digital life but enriches it.

Furthermore, it's essential to teach and practice boundary-setting. The digital world often blurs lines between work, social interaction, and personal time. By setting clear boundaries, we protect our energies, ensuring we're fully present when engaging with others. It could mean setting tech-free times during the day or designating spaces within our home or life that are preserved for personal interaction without the intrusion of digital devices.

In the endeavor to prioritize meaningful connections, gratitude plays a vital role. Regularly acknowledging and appreciating the relationships we cherish strengthens these bonds. A simple "thank you" or a note of appreciation can work wonders. Expressing gratitude fosters a cycle of positivity and goodwill, enriching our interactions and reinforcing meaningful connections.

In conclusion, while the digital age presents unique challenges for maintaining meaningful connections, it simultaneously offers unprecedented opportunities for us to forge and sustain them. Whether through prioritizing quality over quantity, setting boundaries, embracing authenticity, or fostering gratitude, we possess the capability to shape a digital lifestyle that enhances rather than hinders our personal relationships. Let's embrace this challenge, craft our paths thoughtfully, and fill our lives with connections that truly matter.

Crafting a Customized Digital Plan

In our ever-connected world, transforming how we interact with technology begins with crafting a customized digital plan. This plan isn't one-size-fits-all; it's as unique as each person navigating the vast digital landscape. Embracing the idea that digital life can be tailored is empowering in itself. Let's break down how you can create a plan that aligns with your values and enhances your life.

Start by reflecting on what truly matters to you. Are there digital habits that resonate with your core values, or are they more aligned with what others expect from you? Acknowledging this difference is crucial. Consider what aspects of your digital life bring joy and value versus those that drain your energy. It's okay to have diverse experiences online, but intentionality is key. By identifying the elements that serve your goals and aspirations, you craft a path toward a balanced tech life.

Once your priorities are clear, it's time to observe your current digital habits. Keep a log of your online activities for a week. Don't judge yourself harshly; merely observe with curiosity. Which platforms and activities consume your time? What leaves you feeling fulfilled and what leaves you feeling empty? This self-awareness becomes the foundation upon which to build your customized plan.

With insights in hand, it's essential to set specific, achievable goals. These goals serve as the compass for your digital journey. They could include reducing screen time, fostering deeper online connections, or perhaps improving productivity through mindful tech use. Whatever they may be, ensure they are realistic and adaptable. A good plan is like a living document, constantly evolving as your needs and circumstances change.

Consider establishing boundaries that serve as guardrails for your digital life. Just as cities have zoning laws, you can create digital zones in your life. Allocate tech-free times, like during meals or before bedtime, to encourage meaningful offline interactions. Remember, these boundaries are not restrictions; they are permissions to engage in life more fully.

Technology itself can be a tool for balance. Explore apps and tools designed to enhance productivity and mindfulness. Calendar apps can organize your time efficiently, while meditation apps promote calmness and focus. Choose tools that align with your objectives, and don't hesitate to experiment until you find what works best. The trick is to ensure they assist rather than dictate your schedule, helping to maintain the serenity of your plan.

A customized digital plan might include periods of full disconnection, like digital detox days or breaks. These aren't about deprivation; they're about rejuvenation. Disconnecting allows time for introspection and engagement with the physical world around you.

Blocking out times to unplug can deepen your appreciation for the online world when you return, having refreshed your perspective.

Collaborate with friends or family members on this journey. Sharing goals with others not only provides accountability but also offers a support network. Collective digital planning can be enriching, making the journey more joyful and less isolating. Opening conversations about digital habits builds a community of intentional tech users who uplift each other.

Continual reevaluation is essential. A thriving digital plan adapts as life evolves. Regularly assess what's working and what isn't. This approach ensures that the plan remains relevant, fostering growth and balance. As you progress, you'll find greater peace and purpose in your digital interactions.

Crafting a customized digital plan is a pivotal step toward creating a balanced digital life. It's about taking command of your digital journey and making conscious decisions that harmonize with your vision for a fulfilling life. Embrace the process as an opportunity to reconnect with what's important. In doing so, you'll not only gain more control over your digital existence but also find that elusive sense of focus and tranquility in the digital age.

Chapter 8:
Building Digital Resilience

In our fast-paced digital world, building resilience isn't just a luxury—it's a necessity. Digital resilience involves cultivating the ability to navigate the relentless stream of information and distractions with intentionality and grace. It's about developing strategies to manage technology-induced stress and nurturing a relationship with our devices that enhances rather than detracts from our well-being. This means setting boundaries that protect our peace, re-evaluating habits that feed anxiety, and intentionally choosing tech interactions that align with our values. By strengthening our digital resilience, we can transform the overwhelming noise into a harmonious symphony that supports a balanced and fulfilling life.

Coping Strategies for Tech Overwhelm

In a world where technology is ever-present, feeling overwhelmed is hardly unusual. Many of us are caught in a constant cycle of notifications, screens, and digital noise. But this doesn't have to be our reality. By developing coping strategies, we can reclaim a simpler, more focused life where technology serves us, not the other way around.

One of the most powerful strategies is to begin with **mindful awareness**. This involves noticing when technology is causing discomfort or stress. Recognizing these moments is the first step towards change. When you feel that familiar strain in your eyes or a tightening in your chest, pause. Acknowledge that these symptoms are signals from your body, a reminder to step back and reevaluate your tech usage. This moment of pause can transition into an opportunity for reflection and adjustment.

Another strategy to combat tech overwhelm is to *establish clear boundaries*. This means setting time limits on your screen usage and being intentional about when and how you engage with devices. Consider establishing "tech-free zones" or times, such as during meals or the first and last hours of your day. These spaces and times can become sacred, offering a respite for your overworked mind. By creating these boundaries, you encourage a healthier relationship with technology.

Engaging in **alternative activities** is also beneficial. Find joy in offline pursuits like reading, hiking, or engaging in creative endeavors. These activities not only provide a much-needed break from screens but also enrich your life, offering new perspectives and inspirations. By diversifying your activities, you strengthen your ability to cope with tech overwhelm and tap into your creativity.

Connection with others is paramount. In an age of digital interaction, we must not underestimate the power of face-to-face communication. Make a conscious effort to connect with friends, family, or colleagues in person. Meaningful human interaction is an antidote to the superficial connections often cultivated online. Sharing experiences in real-time with others fosters a sense of belonging and helps to anchor you amid the digital swirl.

Another strategy involves **developing a personalized plan** for your digital life. Assess your tech habits and identify which areas bring value and which contribute to overwhelm. Tailor your digital engagement to prioritize what's meaningful to you. For instance, if social media is a source of stress, consider trimming your lists or setting strict time limits. By customizing your digital existence, you exercise control and reduce unnecessary noise.

Practicing self-compassion during this journey is crucial. Understand that setbacks may occur, and that's okay. Change is difficult and progress often involves trial and error. Approach each day as a new opportunity to live more intentionally and to forge a healthier relationship with technology. Be gentle with yourself, and celebrate small victories as you move towards greater digital serenity.

It's also helpful to explore **mindfulness practices** that can be seamlessly incorporated into your routine. Techniques such as meditation or simple breathing exercises can be grounding, providing clarity and calm in a world of constant stimulation. Randomly punctuate your day with these practices to enhance focus and reduce stress. With consistent practice, mindfulness becomes a reliable tool to counteract tech-induced overwhelm.

Digitally detoxing at regular intervals can serve as a reset for your mind and body. Consider dedicating one day a week to disconnect from all screens. Use this time to connect with nature, journal your thoughts, or simply enjoy the peace that comes from unplugging. Regular detoxes remind us of the simplicity and joy found in offline living.

Finally, **educate yourself** about the seductive design components of tech. Knowing how apps and websites are engineered to capture your attention empowers you to make informed choices about your tech use. Build awareness of these techniques to resist the pull of endless scrolling and notifications.

Embracing these coping strategies doesn't mean rejecting technology altogether. Instead, it's about creating a balanced approach where we harness technology's benefits while safeguarding our mental well-being. It's a journey toward digital resilience, where technology enhances, rather than overwhelms, our lives.

By weaving these strategies into our daily routines, we construct a healthier, more intentional engagement with technology. As we master this balance, we find more room for creativity, productivity, and the simple joys of life that often go unnoticed amidst the digital din.

Fostering a Healthy Relationship with Technology

In our fast-paced digital era, fostering a healthy relationship with technology is not just a recommendation; it's essential for maintaining our mental well-being and overall life satisfaction. Many of us might've heard the whispers of digital fatigue, felt the anxiety bubbling up as notifications ding incessantly, or perhaps watched precious hours slip away in the abyss of endless scrolling. Yet, amidst this whirlwind, a harmonious relationship with technology can transform our day-to-day experiences into something richer and more meaningful.

The first step towards nurturing this healthy dynamic is acknowledging that while technology is a powerful tool, it doesn't define us. It's very easy to become wrapped up in the digital ecosystem, equating our self-worth with likes or online achievements. Yet, these digital metrics often miss the depth of our real-world value and capabilities. Instead of letting technology dictate our pace, let's approach it with intentionality, focusing on how it can enhance our lives rather than control them.

Understanding the emotional triggers associated with technology use is crucial. Have you ever noticed a rise in stress when an unread message pops up, or a feeling of inadequacy when a friend's perfect life flashes across your feed? These reactions are normal, yet they signal areas that may require reflection and adjustment. Reflecting on these interactions can shine a light on patterns that need changing. For instance, consider setting boundaries on your social media use during times when you're vulnerable to comparison or anxiety, such as early mornings or late at night.

Building a healthier tech relationship also involves practicing digital mindfulness. This isn't about abstaining from tech but engaging with it in a deliberate and thoughtful way. Instead of multitasking across screens, try focusing on one task at a time. This singular focus not only improves productivity but can also elevate the joy found in the task itself. By being present in our digital interactions, whether we're watching a film, reading an article, or catching up with a friend over video chat, we deepen our engagement and derive more satisfaction.

A practical component of fostering this relationship includes tailoring our tech use to align with our values and intentions. Think of your ideal day: What digital tools genuinely contribute to it? What platforms or apps provide genuine value, and which ones lead to endless rabbit holes? Answering these questions helps in crafting a tech routine that serves your interests and aspirations. Remember, there's no one-size-fits-all approach; it's about what feels right for you.

This journey towards a healthier tech relationship also invites us to pause and savor those moments away from screens. What joys lie in the tactile pleasures of analog experiences? Whether it's the feel of a paper book between your fingers, the rustle of leaves on a nature walk, or the vibrant hues of a painting in progress, these moments bring a profound richness that digital experiences might not capture. By balancing our screen time with these offline pleasures, we embrace a fuller spectrum of experiences.

For many, the workplace presents its own set of challenges. Technology promises efficiency, yet it frequently tempts us toward distraction. Authentic connections with colleagues risk becoming secondary to managing a flood of emails and constant pings. Establishing clear boundaries, such as scheduled blocks for focused work without digital interruptions, can be transformative. By reclaiming control over our tech-led environments, we're not just surviving in the workplace—we're thriving.

Moreover, a balanced digital life benefits not just us but our relationships too. When we model healthy tech habits, it encourages those around us to reflect on their technology use. This can foster a community of intentional tech users who support and inspire one another. Being present during in-person interactions—putting away screens and truly listening—is a bonding gesture and reinforces the message that our relationships are more than just pixels on a screen.

Another pillar of this relationship is resilience. Digital resilience involves adapting to the inevitable changes and challenges that arise in our high-tech lives. Whether it's coping with an unexpected tech malfunction or navigating the constant evolution of platforms, viewing these challenges as opportunities to learn and grow is empowering. Developing a robust toolkit of coping strategies ensures we can mitigate the downsides of our digital lives and increase our capacity to thrive within them.

The road to fostering a healthy relationship with technology is ongoing, requiring regular reflection and adjustments. It's about striving for balance and understanding that while technology plays a significant role in our lives, it shouldn't overshadow the non-digital moments that bring us joy and fulfillment. By actively shaping our tech interactions, we're not only building digital resilience; we're crafting a life that's authentically ours—a life where technology serves us, not the other way around.

Chapter 9:
The Art of Digital Decluttering

In the quest for a serene digital landscape, understanding and tackling digital clutter becomes crucial. Like clearing a messy desk or organizing a chaotic room, digital decluttering is about conscious pruning of what's unnecessary, outdated, or distracting. As our devices overflow with apps, notifications, and files, each piece vying for our attention, the mental burden can become overwhelming. The art lies in uncovering what truly adds value and supports our goals, creating digital spaces that breathe clarity and focus. It's an ongoing process, not a one-time task, where intentional choices and mindful sorting lead to a cleaner, more intentional digital life. Embracing this practice frees us from the weight of digital noise, making space for creativity, peace, and a deeper connection with our priorities. So, let yourself embark on this liberating journey of letting go, and witness the transformative power of a simplified digital realm.

Identifying Digital Clutter

In a world where digital devices have become extensions of ourselves, identifying digital clutter is essential for finding balance and clarity. Just like our physical spaces can become overwhelmed with possessions, our digital realms are prone to accumulation. This clutter, though intangible, has a profound impact on our mental well-being, productivity, and overall peace of mind.

Start by asking yourself: What does digital clutter mean to you? For many, it's those countless unread emails, a photo gallery filled with identical shots, or apps downloaded impulsively but rarely used. It's those browser tabs left open, promising a later return that never comes. Digital clutter isn't limited to just files and apps; it encompasses all the unnecessary digital noise consuming our attention without adding any significant value to our lives.

Recognizing digital clutter demands an honest audit of how we spend our time online. Have you ever noticed how much time slips away while scrolling through endless social media feeds, attending to emails, or browsing aimlessly? The digital world is meticulously designed to captivate us, often leading to the accumulation of clutter that we don't even perceive accumulating.

Think about your devices. Every app, document, or notification that doesn't serve a purpose contributes to this clutter. Each digital interaction carries a weight that demands our mental resources. We find ourselves mentally taxed, not necessarily because of one task but because of the sum of all these accumulated digital interactions. It's here that identifying digital clutter becomes crucial to our mental clarity and emotional balance.

But how can we distinguish between essential and cluttered digital interactions? Start by categorizing your digital activities into priorities, obligations, and distractions. Priorities are interactions that add value or joy, such as connecting meaningfully with loved ones or learning something new. Obligations are tasks that demand our attention but aren't necessarily fulfilling. Distractions are those mindless pursuits that lead us down a rabbit hole without any conscious decision.

This categorization may be challenging. We often confuse obligations with priorities, thinking that being constantly available online is essential to our roles at work or in our personal lives.

However, not all obligations are truly essential, and recognizing this distinction is crucial.

Equally important is acknowledging that digital clutter is subjective. What feels overwhelming to one person might be perfectly manageable to another. The key is emotional resonance. Ask yourself how each digital interaction makes you feel. Do your online activities leave you feeling exhausted, or do they invigorate you? This self-assessment forms the backbone of identifying and subsequently reducing digital clutter.

To effectively identify digital clutter, begin with a digital detox exercise. Dedicate a period, perhaps a weekend, to consciously reduce your digital interactions. Track what you miss and what you don't. Often, this exercise will reveal surprising insights, highlighting interactions you thought were priorities but actually provided little value to your well-being.

Remember, the goal isn't merely to eliminate everything but to discern what truly matters. Embrace the concept of intentionality. Each app you open, every notification you check, should be a conscious choice. This shift from autopilot to intentionality is the crux of reducing digital clutter and reclaiming your mental space.

Another strategy is to periodically review your digital spaces. Just as you might declutter your home every season, apply the same principle to your digital environment. Organize your files, delete unnecessary apps, and clean out your inbox. Make this a routine practice, integrating it into your lifestyle rather than viewing it as a one-time task.

Additionally, consider the architecture of your digital world. Are your devices configured to support your intentional use, or do they inadvertently contribute to your clutter? Simplifying your digital layout can go a long way in preventing unnecessary distractions. This might mean reducing the immediacy of notifications, curating your app collection, or even restructuring your home screen to reflect what truly matters.

Empathy towards oneself during this process is vital. It's easy to get frustrated with your initial habits or the seeming impossibility of managing digital clutter effectively. But remember, digital clutter is a societal issue, born out of the digital age's conveniences and complexities. We are bombarded with options, and no one is immune to the lure of incessant connectivity.

As you navigate this digital decluttering journey, be gentle with yourself. Celebrate small victories—a cleaned-up folder, a deleted app, a weekend spent offline. Each step you take towards reducing digital clutter brings you closer to a more mindful and fulfilling relationship with technology. While technology can be a powerful ally, its benefits are best harnessed with intentional use, allowing us to focus on what truly enriches our lives.

In conclusion, identifying digital clutter is a pivotal step in the art of digital decluttering. By understanding its nuanced presence in our daily lives, we can begin to reconfigure our relationship with technology, fostering a space that supports our focus and enhances our well-being. This journey requires patience and persistence, but each effort you make brings you closer to a life where technology is a tool for growth and connection, not a source of overwhelm.

Implementing a Decluttering Plan

In today's whirlwind of digital chaos, finding clarity might seem like a distant dream. Yet, beneath the notifications and emails, there's a realm where simplicity reigns—not unlike the tranquil feeling of a well-organized room. Implementing a digital decluttering plan is your gateway to this serene space. You're not just tidying up pixels but reclaiming your mental space, which has been hijacked by bits and bytes, one notification at a time.

The journey begins with awareness. It's crucial to first recognize what constitutes digital clutter in your life. Is it the unread newsletters piling up in your inbox, or the chaos of unorganized bookmarks? Perhaps it's the endless apps downloaded—but rarely used—that fill your phone storage. Each of these is a stealthy thief of focus and peace. Identify them clearly and intentionally; this is your first step in removing their unwelcome presence.

Once you've identified the digital clutter, the next move involves prioritization. Not all digital clutter is created equal. Some items demand immediate attention, while others can remain on the back burner. Start with a list—prioritization empowers you to tackle what's most disruptive to your mental clarity first. By dealing with the loudest noise, you create a ripple effect of tranquility throughout your digital landscape.

As you categorize, ask yourself probing questions: "Does this digital clutter add value?" "Does it enhance my life or merely keep my thumbs busy?" By intentionally questioning the necessity of each component, you're paving the way toward a mindful and intentional digital presence. This step may feel reminiscent of Marie Kondo's philosophy—if it doesn't spark joy or utility, it should be let go.

Next comes the phase of action. This is where you physically—or digitally—begin the removal process. Unsubscribe, delete, and organize with fanfare. Let your inbox breathe by unsubscribing from newsletters that no longer serve you. Your discretion is a precious resource; guard it well by choosing to retain digital items that contribute positively to your life.

The purge might feel daunting, almost like a digital baptism of sorts, but take heart in knowing that it's a step towards liberation. It isn't about creating a blank slate but rather a curated digital environment that encourages focus and creativity. A cleaned-up desktop, organized folders, and a decluttered phone screen can become beacons of clarity rather than sources of stress and confusion.

Digital decluttering isn't a one-time event but an ongoing practice—like weeding a garden, recurrent maintenance prevents overwhelming growth. Establish a routine for regular clean-ups. You might find that a monthly digital sweep aligns well with your rhythm. Set aside time to reassess digital content and ensure your online environment aligns with your current goals and values.

Consider implementing a regular "digital sabbatical." A day or a weekend of complete disconnection can reframe your perspective and remind you of the joys beyond the screen. Think of it as hitting a collective home button on your devices and your mind. Stepping back allows you to return with renewed clarity and a sense of purpose.

Another element is cultivating mindful digital habits. Introduce friction to your tech use where it's needed. Simple changes like moving a distracting app off your home screen can act as a gentle reminder to assess whether its use aligns with your intentions at that moment. It's akin to placing hurdles not for obstruction but for mindful deliberation.

Sharing your progress with a community can also provide support and accountability. Like in any decluttering process, there are moments of questioning and overwhelm. A community of like-minded individuals can offer encouragement and new perspectives. Whether it's through online forums or meet-ups, sharing your journey fosters a communal bond over digital minimalism.

Remember, the ultimate aim of digital decluttering is more than just tidying up your tech life; it's about reclaiming your most precious resource—time. The minutes spent on mindless scrolling can be redirected towards hobbies, connections, and experiences that truly matter. The art of digital decluttering, then, isn't solely about subtraction, but about adding depth and meaning into your everyday interactions.

Your decluttered digital space is a testament to your commitment to serenity in the face of digital chaos. As you walk this path, you'll find that each byte you consciously manage contributes not just to your peace of mind, but to your holistic well-being. The destination is a smoother, more intentional interaction with technology, offering you the headspace to focus on what really counts.

In this pursuit, acknowledge the progress you make, however small it may seem. Embrace the freedom that comes from each decision to curate your digital footprint. As the noise fades, what emerges is a clearer, more focused vision of yourself and the technology that supports—not intrudes upon—your life's tapestry.

Chapter 10:
The Role of Social Media

In a world where social media occupies a pivotal space in our digital lives, understanding its impact is crucial for achieving digital harmony. Social media platforms offer unprecedented opportunities for connection and expression, but they can also become sources of distraction and emotional strain. It's essential to evaluate how these platforms fit into our daily routines and mental landscapes. By fostering an intentional approach to social media usage, we can reclaim our focus and well-being. Conscious engagement means actively choosing what content serves our growth and aligning our online interactions with our values. By doing so, we not only mitigate the negative aspects of social media but also harness its potential to enrich our lives, creating a balanced and mindful digital existence.

Evaluating Your Social Media Usage

Social media, a dazzling realm of likes, shares, and endless scrolls, often feels like a double-edged sword. On one hand, it connects us to friends, family, and a world of information at our fingertips. On the other hand, the constant barrage of notifications and pressures to present perfect versions of ourselves can leave us feeling drained. Evaluating your social media habits is a crucial step in reclaiming your sense of peace and focus in an increasingly noisy world.

Begin by asking yourself a simple yet profound question: What do I genuinely seek from my social media experience? Is it a sense of community, a platform for self-expression, or maybe just a convenient way to stay informed? Reflecting on this can reveal whether your current usage aligns with your true intentions. Many times, our scrolling becomes automatic, driven more by habit than by purpose. Identifying this gap is the first step in making intentional adjustments.

Once you've gained clarity on your intentions, take a moment to quantify your usage. How much time do you spend on social media each day? There are various tools and apps available that can help track this. You might find the numbers startling—what felt like just a few minutes may actually add up to hours. Being aware of this can be a wake-up call, urging you to set more conscious limits on your engagement.

Equally important is examining the impact of social media on your mental and emotional well-being. Do you feel uplifted after a session, or do you find yourself comparing your life unfavorably to the curated lives of others? Recognizing emotions such as envy, inadequacy, or anxiety when using social media can help you discern whether it's serving you well or if it's time for a digital detox.

Identifying the specific platforms and interactions that enhance your life versus those that drain it can act as a guide in crafting a more intentional social media experience. For example, connecting with a supportive community discussing mutual interests might be beneficial, while endless scrolling through celebrity gossip might be less so. Understanding the content and connections that positively or negatively affect you allows for a more refined approach to social media use.

Consider the influence of both active and passive engagement in your digital life. Active engagement—commenting lovingly on a friend's post or sharing high-quality content—often feels more rewarding and interactive. Conversely, passive consumption, where you endlessly scroll without interacting, can leave you feeling empty.

Striking a balance between these different types of engagements can significantly enhance your experience and reduce feelings of digital fatigue.

Reducing screen time on social media also involves setting boundaries, both in terms of time and in terms of what you're willing to engage with. Decide specific times of day when you'll check your accounts, perhaps once in the morning and once in the evening. This structure not only gives you more freedom throughout the day, but it also lessens the impulse to check your devices continuously.

Moreover, implementing content filters or unfollowing accounts that consistently bring negativity into your life is crucial. Curating a feed that inspires, educates, and entertains in a healthy way can transform social media from a source of stress into an asset. Remember, you have control over what you allow into your digital space.

As you reflect on these practices, it's important to stay compassionate with yourself. Changing habits, especially those reinforced by the dopamine hits of likes and shares, isn't easy. It's a journey of small, deliberate steps that can lead to a more mindful and fulfilling engagement with technology.

Reevaluating your social media usage isn't about complete elimination—it's about transformation. By navigating these online spaces with purpose and intention, you can find a balance that respects your time and serves your true desires. In doing so, these tools can once again become what they were meant to be: sources of connection, joy, and community, rather than distraction and anxiety. The key lies in consistently aligning your digital actions with your values, creating a digital environment that supports rather than undermines your goals.

Strategies for Conscious Engagement

Engaging with social media consciously is akin to navigating a bustling cityscape. If you're not deliberate, you'll find yourself distracted by every flashy billboard and noise. Social media, a powerful tool in our digital age, offers us unparalleled opportunities for connection and information. Yet, left unchecked, it can also lead to feelings of overwhelm and disconnection from reality. The goal is to harness its benefits while minimizing its pitfalls through intentional, mindful engagement.

Understanding the platforms we use is the first step towards conscious engagement. Each social media platform is designed with algorithms that leverage our attention. By learning how these algorithms function, we can start using these platforms without being used by them. For instance, both Facebook and Instagram serve content based on past engagement, perpetuating a cycle of endless scrolling. Being aware of this allows us to take back control and decide which content genuinely enriches our lives.

Next, setting boundaries with social media is crucial. Have you ever found yourself picking up your phone, meaning to just check a couple of notifications, only to realize an hour has slipped by? Establishing clear limits can prevent such spirals. Consider allocating specific times in your day for social media use, akin to how you would schedule a meeting or a workout. Over time, these deliberate boundaries can transform your relationship with your digital devices, providing more time for other fulfilling activities.

Equally important is the practice of curating your social media feeds intentionally. Consider what types of content leave you feeling inspired, informed, or connected. Is it the news updates, friends' life events, or motivational content? Unfollow or mute accounts that consistently drain your energy and focus on those that add value. This selective approach not only reduces digital chaos but also ensures your time online aligns with your personal values.

Moreover, engaging consciously requires regular reflection on how social media affects your mood and behavior. After spending time online, pause to assess your emotional state. Are you feeling inspired, anxious, content, or envious? Recognizing these emotions can guide you in adjusting your interaction patterns. Over time, this self-awareness cultivates a healthier approach to digital interactions, allowing you to enjoy the benefits of social media without sacrificing your mental equilibrium.

Developing digital mindfulness is another key strategy. This involves being present in your actions and interactions online. It means engaging with content and people actively rather than passively consuming information. When you're scrolling through posts, practice stopping to think about your reactions and responses. Comment with intention, share information with discernment, and engage in discussions with an open mind. Each of these steps encourages purposeful and rewarding social interactions.

Incorporating breaks or a social media detox can further enhance your engagement strategy. Taking time away from social media, even just for a day, can refresh your perspective and lessen dependency. During these breaks, find alternative activities that nurture your well-being. This could be reading a book, going for a walk, or spending quality time with loved ones without digital distractions. These pauses can remind us of the joys present in offline life, fostering a healthier balance between our digital and physical worlds.

Community involvement can also amplify the benefits of social media. Look for communities that motivate and support you towards positive change. Engage with groups and pages dedicated to interests, hobbies, or causes you're passionate about. Not only does this create a supportive network of like-minded individuals, but it also transforms your online presence into a platform for personal growth and development.

Lastly, cultivating an attitude of gratitude in your online interactions can shift your focus from consumption to contribution. By appreciating and acknowledging the positive aspects of your digital communities, you enhance the meaningfulness of your interactions. Express thanks for the content that influences you positively, celebrate achievements shared by others, and contribute your own stories and insights. This practice not only enriches your experience but also amplifies positivity within the digital spheres you inhabit.

In conclusion, social media isn't inherently good or bad; it's a tool that reflects our intentions. By consciously engaging with these platforms, setting boundaries, curating content, and practicing mindfulness, we can transform a potential source of anxiety into one of inspiration and connection. It's about making deliberate choices that align with our values and encourage well-being. As we navigate the digital landscape with purpose, we reclaim our attention, foster deeper connections, and create space for peace in a world often cluttered with noise.

Chapter 11:
Managing Notifications and Interruptions

In our quest for a balanced digital life, managing notifications and interruptions is a crucial step towards reclaiming focus and peace. Today's world, buzzing with alerts and pings, can easily pull us away from meaningful tasks. But what if we took a different approach? Customizing alerts allows us to filter the noise, letting only the truly important messages break through. This isn't about ignoring the world—it's about choosing when and how it engages with us. Techniques like batching notifications, using "Do Not Disturb" settings, and scheduling specific times for checking messages can reduce constant disruptions, fostering a calmer, more deliberate interaction with technology. By doing so, we invite space for creativity and thoughtfulness, carving a path towards a more intentional and fulfilling use of our devices. Let us embrace the art of interruption management as a transformative practice that enhances not just our productivity, but the quality of our lives as well.

Customizing Alerts for Peace

In our hyper-connected world, alerts and notifications have become omnipresent, constantly vying for our attention. These seemingly innocuous pings, beeps, and vibrations can cumulatively contribute to a heightened sense of anxiety and overwhelm. Yet, with thoughtful customization, alerts can transition from being a source of interruption to a serene aspect of your digital life. The goal is to reclaim control over your notifications to foster an environment conducive to peace, focus, and well-being.

Imagine you're deeply immersed in a task, and suddenly, a notification breaks the flow. It's a random update, perhaps not even relevant to your current priorities. This interruption not only derails your train of thought but also fragments your cognitive engagement. According to researchers, it can take upwards of 20 minutes to refocus fully after such a disruption. The good news is, by consciously managing your alerts, you can minimize these distractions significantly.

Start by conducting an audit of your current notification settings across devices. Enlist the help of focus-enhancing methods such as setting aside time to review which apps truly deserve your immediate attention and which can wait. Many of us retain the default notification settings, which are often designed to maximize app engagement rather than safeguard your serenity. Differentiate between alerts that are necessary for your professional responsibilities and those that are merely habitual intrusions. Customization is key.

Consider creating tiers of notifications. For instance, critical messages from family or work may remain audible, while less urgent updates silently accumulate until you choose to address them. By honing in on what truly matters, you're establishing a digital boundary that aligns with your personal and professional values. This mindful approach to technology helps reinforce that you're in charge, rather than at the whim of every ping and buzz.

Visualize your most serene environment—whether a quiet nook at home or a calm bench in a leafy park. Strive to emulate this sense of tranquility in your digital space by leveraging "Do Not Disturb" settings or scheduling notification-free times during peak productivity or relaxation hours. Remember, these settings can often be adjusted not just globally, but app-by-app, ensuring a bespoke balance between accessibility and peace.

Empower yourself with the knowledge of app-specific benefits. Many apps now offer "silent" notifications that appear without sound, reducing their potential to disturb. Others provide "digest" options, compiling alerts into a single notification delivered at a preset interval. Using these tools thoughtfully can help streamline the information you're bombarded with, ensuring that only critical updates interrupt your mental peace.

Reflect on how you react to notifications. The compelling urge to address every alert may need to be consciously unlearned. Part of customizing for peace is altering your interaction style— acknowledging that not every incoming alert demands immediate action. This gives room for cultivating a more deliberate relationship with your technology. If you're uncomfortable ignoring some notifications, experiment with setting specific check-in times to review them.

Remember, the aim isn't to disconnect entirely, but to foster a deliberate connection. The richness of life isn't in the bountiful info stream; rather, it may lie in the deeper understanding and purposeful action nurtured through mindful presence and engagement. By getting to grips with your digital alerts, you'll be creating space for moments of clarity and insight—to not only hear but to truly listen to the nuances of both your digital and real-world surroundings.

Inventive self-awareness in managing alerts not only nurtures peace but also drives personal and professional growth. A tranquil digital environment doesn't form overnight. But by leaning into the adjustment process, tweaking settings, and revisiting choices often, you'll craft a space that supports calmness and efficacy. As you dedicate time to refining these digital boundaries, recognize that you're paving the way toward a more intentional, fulfilling relationship with technology.

Turning notifications from noise to melody requires an ongoing commitment to change. Expect the need to reevaluate as life shifts, as what works in one phase may not in another. Stay attuned to how changes affect you—emotionally and productivity-wise. With a bit of self-examination, you can continually fine-tune your digital world to echo the priorities of your innermost values.

As you navigate this path, know that peace is not merely the absence of interferences but the presence of something profound: a balance. Through customization, you're not only adjusting settings but shaping your digital landscape to be one of harmony, so that every interaction resonates with meaning, cutting through the noise to enhance your life.

Techniques for Reducing Interruptions

In our hyper-connected world, interruptions are a constant companion, persistently vying for our attention and eroding our focus. Yet, the quest for a harmonious digital life necessitates that we learn to manage these interruptions effectively. There are practical, empowering techniques which can be adopted to lessen distractions and foster a space where concentration can flourish. Embracing these techniques doesn't imply shutting out the world entirely but creating a buffer that allows you to engage with the digital sphere on your terms.

Start by scrutinizing the sources of your interruptions. Emails, notifications, app alerts—they all demand our immediate attention, pulling us away from tasks at hand. By auditing these stimuli, you gain clarity over which are truly critical and which are merely noise. This inventory acts as the foundation upon which to build a more focused digital environment. It's not about drowning out the world but selecting which whispers you choose to follow.

Once you've identified the prime interrupters, it's time to customize your digital interfaces to diminish their impact. Adjusting settings on your devices to control when and how you receive notifications can drastically cut down on unexpected distractions. For instance, enabling "Do Not Disturb" modes during peak productivity hours allows for a protected window of concentration. While this may seem a simple measure, the real triumph lies in reclaiming ownership over your attention and time.

Another powerful technique is the strategic scheduling of regular intervals for checking messages and notifications. Instead of constantly reacting to each ping or buzz, designate specific times to engage with these communications. This not only helps in preserving your focus but also trains your mind to concentrate on tasks uninterrupted. It's a subtle shift with profound implications for productivity and mental peace.

Physical space also plays a pivotal role in how we manage interruptions. Creating a deliberate workspace that minimizes digital distractions can significantly enhance focus. Consider the placement of devices like smartphones, which are often the primary source of interruptions. Keeping them out of reach or even out of sight can prevent the habitual glance or reach that breaks your concentration. Such physical adjustments complement digital strategies and reinforce an environment conducive to deep work.

It's essential to cultivate awareness of our cognitive rhythms and listen to when we are most prone to distractions. Some find their attention waning in the afternoons, while others struggle with focus in the morning. Recognizing these patterns allows us to tailor our approach: scheduling high-interruption tasks during these vulnerable periods and reserving demanding work for times when focus naturally peaks.

Moreover, mindfulness practices can serve as a shield against interruptions. Techniques like meditation and deep breathing enhance our ability to maintain calm and redirect attention effectively when distractions arise. Regular practice of these techniques doesn't just build resistance to interruptions but enriches overall well-being, making them a cornerstone of a balanced digital life.

Incorporating physical movement or brief interludes of silence into your daily routine can also recalibrate focus and eliminate interruption fatigue. Such breaks don't detract from productivity; they renew it. A short walk, some outdoor air, or even mindful stretching can act as a powerful reset, allowing you to return to work refreshed and less susceptible to distractions.

Furthermore, leverage digital tools purpose-built to bolster focus and limit interruptions. Apps designed to lock distracting sites or track time allow you to set boundaries on your digital engagement. These tools act as allies, reinforcing your intention and discipline to maintain focus in the face of persistent digital noise. However, it's critical to choose these aids intentionally, ensuring they align with personal needs rather than adding another layer of complexity.

Another often overlooked strategy involves cultivating a culture of respect for uninterrupted time both personally and professionally. Open dialogues with colleagues and loved ones set expectations about availability and periods of focused work. This cultural shift can foster an environment where undisturbed focus is valued and protected, promoting mutual understanding and respect for each other's need for concentration.

Finally, periodically reassessing and refining your approach to handling interruptions is crucial. As technology evolves, so do our habits and the challenges they present. Regular reflection allows us to adapt to new circumstances, ensuring that our strategies for managing interruptions remain relevant and effective. This ongoing commitment to adjustment exemplifies a dynamic and resilient approach to digital life management.

Incorporating these techniques into your daily routine not only mitigates the incessant interruptions but celebrates your autonomy over your digital interactions. It empowers you to design a life that prioritizes mental clarity and focus, setting the stage for a mindful engagement with technology. As you experiment with these strategies, remember that the journey towards reduced interruptions is personal and iterative, evolving as you reshape your digital landscape.

Chapter 12:
Embracing Analog Alternatives

As we stand at the crossroads of a digital-dominated culture, the path to tranquility often lies in rediscovering the analog pleasures that once filled our days. It's not merely about stepping away from screens, but about immersing ourselves in activities that reconnect us with the tangible world. Whether it's delving into the pages of a book or savoring the tactile experience of crafting something by hand, these pursuits remind us of the simplicity and joy found in the offline realm. Embracing such activities can serve as a balm for the digital burnout so many of us feel. In finding balance with technology, we pave the way for meaningful engagement with our surroundings, fostering a renewed sense of peace and fulfillment. This shift is not about rejecting technology altogether, but rather choosing mindful moments where the analog reclaims its rightful space in our lives, allowing us to breathe, reflect, and thrive with a more serene mind.

The Joy of Offline Activities

In a world where digital devices continually clamor for our attention, offline activities stand as vital refuges that offer solace and clarity. These activities, unencumbered by screens or buzzing notifications, invite us into spaces of contemplation and creativity. It's through offline activities that we often find ourselves reconnecting with the slower, more deliberate rhythms of life, which, in turn, rejuvenate our weary minds.

Imagine a morning spent perusing a local farmer's market. Here, among the colorful displays of fruits and vegetables, you're transported into a sensory experience that's rich and grounding. The vibrant hues, the intricate textures, the earthy smells—all of these details meld into a symphony that digital experiences can't replicate. Participants exchange genuine conversations, filled with warmth and humor, rather than succinct text messages. In these exchanges, connection feels immediate and real.

An afternoon in a park, with a blanket stretched out beneath sprawling trees, embodies another layer of offline joy. As the sun filters through branches and plays upon the pages of a book, engrossment replaces scattered thoughts brought on by multitasking screens. Reading becomes a meditative act, allowing deep focus and an immersion into worlds that feel unrushed and expansive. Unlike digital skimming, the pages of a book invite us to linger on words and ideas, to savor the beauty of language itself.

Consider the rhythmic strokes of painting or the feel of knitting needles in your hands—each offers a tactile connection that our devices can't provide. These activities slow time, encouraging a measured pace that lets creativity unfold naturally. Rather than swiping through endless feeds, creating with physical materials develops patience and persistence. The end result is more than just a finished product; it is a testament to taking the time to immerse oneself in the act of creation.

Music, too, has a profound offline life. When playing an instrument or attending a live concert, sound becomes an avenue of expression and connection. A live performance, with its unique energy and interactions between musicians and audience, creates a shared experience distinct from listening through earbuds. The ebb and flow of rhythm and melody capture emotion in ways that transcend the digital realm, fostering a shared sense of presence and aliveness.

Gardening is another delightful offline pursuit, and it provides a direct link to nature's cycles and rhythms. Tending to plants means cultivating patience and nurturing growth over time. The feel of soil, the sound of rustling leaves, and the sight of sprouting seeds connect us to the Earth's vast ecosystems. Whether you tend a sprawling garden or a modest collection of potted plants, the joy in seeing life burgeon under your care goes beyond what can be experienced through a screen.

In a digital-centric world, offline activities help anchor us in the present moment. These pursuits remind us to engage deeply with the physical world and foster a mindfulness that cultivates peace and presence. In these moments of engagement, we recognize the richness of life untethered to pixels. Each offline activity becomes a practice in being, drawing our attention away from the noise of the digital and towards the nuances of our immediate surroundings.

Engaging in offline activities isn't about rejecting technology but about restoring balance. It's about making conscious choices to allocate time and energy to experiences that nourish the soul. Perhaps it's drawing a bath and letting the warmth and quiet wash over you. Or maybe it's hiking along a familiar trail, where the bird calls and rustling leaves form a natural symphony. These activities do more than distract—they enrich and ground us, fostering a connection to ourselves and others that feels genuine and enduring.

In embracing offline activities, we open ourselves to a wealth of experiences that are as varied as they are fulfilling. From writing letters to cooking meals from scratch, these pursuits allow us to express individuality and creativity in ways platforms can't capture. They represent a reclaiming of time, encouraging us to engage fully in each moment and cultivate a life that's lived, not just viewed through a screen.

The joy of offline activities is found in their simplicity and depth. These experiences invite us to lose ourselves and discover something authentic and profound. As you navigate your own journey through digital minimalism, consider how these offline activities can serve as both an escape and a return—a return to the essence of what it means to live fully and with intention.

Rediscovering Hobbies and Passions

In today's fast-paced, digital-driven world, it's easy to forget the simple joys that come from engaging in hobbies. These activities not only offer a respite from our glowing screens but also allow us to cultivate skills, patience, and creativity. While digital entertainment is accessible and often immersive, rediscovering hobbies of the past can be an anchor, grounding us amidst the whirlwind of notifications and digital noise.

Imagine the quiet satisfaction of completing a complex jigsaw puzzle. It's an exercise in patience, requiring us to slow down and focus intently on the task at hand. Moreover, these moments allow our minds a chance to wander freely, unburdened by the relentless barrage of email alerts and social media updates. These spaces for daydreaming and introspection are crucial for mental well-being and are often lost in a hyper-connected lifestyle.

Consider the art of crafting, whether it's knitting a scarf, painting a landscape, or building a model airplane. These activities not only engage our hands but also demand a level of mindful presence that many of us have lost in our daily rush. They require attention to detail and an appreciation for the process rather than the outcome. In essence, they teach us to value the journey and find pleasure in the present moment.

Many find solace in rekindling their love for musical instruments. Sitting down at a piano or picking up a guitar can be an emotional release, a form of expression that doesn't rely on the validation of likes or followers but rather creates an intimate dialogue between the musician and their instrument. The same could be said for dance or playing a sport, where the body becomes a vehicle for releasing stress, creating a sensation of freedom and vitality that's hard to replicate in any digital medium.

Gardening is another analog activity that can bring significant joy and satisfaction. There's something profoundly therapeutic about nurturing plants and witnessing their growth over time. It connects us back to the earth, reminding us of the rhythms of nature and our place within it. For many, gardens become sanctuaries where they can momentarily escape the pressures of the digital world and reconnect with life's simplicity and beauty.

Why do these hobbies often feel so rewarding? At the heart of it is the deep sense of autonomy and accomplishment they provide. Unlike the instant gratification of digital feedback loops, hobbies require dedication and offer a reward structure that's more subtle and enriching. They remind us of our agency and capacity to create, build, and solve. In these moments, we reclaim a piece of ourselves that digital culture can sometimes overshadow.

Rediscovering old passions also invites us to explore new interests or skills. Have you ever wanted to learn to cook an elaborate dish or practice calligraphy? These endeavors encourage lifelong learning, instilling a sense of curiosity and purpose that counteracts digital lethargy. They push us outside our comfort zones and cultivate resilience and growth that extend beyond the specific hobby itself.

Group activities, such as joining a book club or a community choir, can provide both the benefit of pursuing a hobby and fostering meaningful human connection. In these settings, we interact face-to-face, share experiences, and connect on deeper levels — aspects often missing in purely digital interactions. It highlights the importance of community and shared experiences that form the backbone of our social well-being.

Nonetheless, reintegrating hobbies into our lives isn't always straightforward. It requires deliberate intention and sometimes effort to carve out time away from screens. One practical approach is to dedicate specific periods in your weekly schedule for hobby activities, just as you'd schedule meetings or other appointments. This intentional time-blocking honors the importance of these pursuits in maintaining a balanced, satisfying life.

Some might feel they've lost touch with what truly ignites their passion or doubt whether it's too late to start something new. But remember, beginning anew isn't a sign of going backward but a testament to your eagerness to evolve and embrace life's diverse experiences. The key lies in approaching these activities with an open heart and mind, ready to accept imperfection and learning curves as part of the process.

Additionally, it's crucial to eliminate the pressure of perfectionism. Your art doesn't need to hang in a gallery, your garden doesn't have to mimic those featured in magazines, and your roasted chicken doesn't have to be a culinary masterpiece. What matters most is the joy and fulfillment you get from the act itself, untainted by external validation.

Rediscovering hobbies and passions can transform how we engage with the world. Free from digital distractions, these analog activities enrich our lives with joy, creativity, and balance. They serve as reminders to cherish the tangible, the tactile, and the rewarding satisfaction that comes from creating and engaging beyond the screen's confines. Let these hobbies be a celebration of slowness and a testament to your journey toward a more intentional, fulfilling relationship with technology and life.

Chapter 13:
Digital Detox for Families

In our fast-paced, tech-driven world, it's crucial for families to carve out spaces and times where technology takes a backseat. Creating family tech rules isn't just about limiting screen time; it's about reconnecting with each other and rediscovering the joy of simple, shared experiences. Encouraging outdoor play and engagement leads to opportunities for children and adults alike to explore, learn, and bond in ways that screens simply can't replicate. Imagine the therapeutic sound of leaves crunching underfoot, the thrill of climbing to the top of a hill, or a simple conversation around a campfire. By making intentional choices to step away from screens, families can foster deeper connections, build resilience, and instill values of presence and mindfulness that benefit not just the household but the broader community too. A digital detox helps create a culture of togetherness and reminds us of the world beyond the screen—a world rich with wonder, conversation, and warmth that nurtures our souls and strengthens our bonds.

Creating Family Tech Rules

In today's digitally saturated world, where screens seem omnipresent, creating family tech rules is not just a suggestion but a necessity. Our homes can become sanctuaries from the perpetual ping of notifications and the relentless scroll of social media feeds. By establishing family tech rules, we can cultivate a nurturing environment that fosters connection, creativity, and presence. These rules serve as a guide, helping families navigate their digital landscapes more mindfully and intentionally.

The first step in crafting family tech rules is collaboration. Involving everyone in the family, regardless of age, ensures a sense of ownership and commitment to the guidelines set. Start by hosting a family meeting where everyone can voice their opinions and concerns about current tech usage. This can be an enlightening exercise, revealing not only the habits each family member has adopted but also their aspirations for a more harmonious relationship with technology.

Establishing clear and realistic boundaries is essential. Set specific times for tech-free interactions, such as during family meals or before bedtime, to promote meaningful conversations and improve sleep quality. These moments, undisturbed by devices, allow families to engage deeply with one another, strengthening bonds and fostering intimacy. Moreover, they create opportunities for reflection, helping individuals process their thoughts and feelings without digital interference.

It is also critical to define acceptable screen time limits based on age and necessity. Understanding that technology is an integral part of modern education and entertainment, balancing its use is crucial. Encourage activities that stimulate creativity and learning, whether it's through educational apps or engaging in family-friendly online games. However, these should be balanced with offline activities, fostering a healthy mix of digital and analog experiences.

While it might feel challenging to enforce these rules, consistency is key. Create visual reminders, like a family tech rule chart, that can be easily referenced. This can function as a constant reminder of the commitment one has made to fostering a healthier digital environment. Such visual tools can also serve as a point of pride and motivation, symbolizing the family's united effort toward digital well-being.

Dialogue is invaluable in this process. Regularly revisit the established rules to assess their effectiveness and relevance. As children grow and technology evolves, adaptations may be necessary. Foster an open environment where family members can express how the rules are impacting them and share suggestions for improvement. This ongoing conversation can cultivate resilience and mutual understanding, ensuring the rules remain dynamic and impactful.

In today's connected age, modeling desired behavior is arguably more influential than the rules themselves. Parents and guardians set the tone for technology use. Practicing what you preach not only reinforces the rules but also instills a sense of integrity and respect within the family. Demonstrating a mindful approach to technology can inspire children to adopt similar habits, reinforcing the values underpinning the family's tech rules.

Finally, create a culture of celebration around the successes of mindful tech use. Recognize and reward times when family members adhere to the tech rules, celebrating the small wins that collectively contribute to the family's digital detox journey. This can be as simple as a verbal acknowledgment or as elaborate as a tech-free family outing. These positive reinforcements can motivate continued adherence to the established norms and foster a supportive atmosphere for growth and learning.

In conclusion, creating family tech rules is a proactive step towards a balanced digital life. By setting boundaries, engaging in open dialogue, and modeling mindful behavior, families can transform their relationship with technology. This chapter of digital detox not only strives for less screen time but for more meaningful, connected, and fulfilling interactions at home. It's a journey that, with commitment and creativity, can yield lifelong benefits for every family member.

Encouraging Outdoor Play and Engagement

Fostering a healthy digital diet for families often begins by stepping outside. Creating opportunities for outdoor play and engagement is not just about keeping the kids entertained; it's about nurturing a profound connection to the natural world that technology, as compelling as it may be, simply can't replicate. Embracing the outdoors invites us to explore a vast and beautiful setting that stimulates all the senses and fosters physical and emotional well-being.

Unstructured outdoor play is essential for children's development. When kids play outside, they engage in physical activities that build strength and coordination. They learn to navigate the world around them, developing critical thinking and problem-solving skills as they assess risks and rewards in real-time. Importantly, outdoor play encourages creativity. A stick can become a sword, a fort, or a makeshift fishing pole, igniting the imagination in ways that digital screens cannot. This creative exploration is vital for developing innovative thinking that benefits them as they grow into adults.

But let's not leave the adults out of the equation. Embracing outdoor activities as a family creates shared experiences that can strengthen bonds. Weekend hiking trips, picnics in the park, or simple backyard games can become cherished traditions that the whole family looks forward to. They create memories that aren't stored as digital files but in the stories we tell and the laughter we share. These moments of genuine presence and engagement help build communication skills and emotional resilience, essential tools for navigating the complexities of today's digital world.

Moreover, nature offers a unique setting for mindfulness, providing a space where one can disconnect from the incessant digital noise and reconnect with oneself. Just taking a stroll in a local park or along a beach can become a meditative practice, allowing thoughts to flow freely, unburdened by alerts or notifications. Here, we can slow down and savor each moment, an antidote to the fast-paced, instantaneous lifestyle that screens often demand.

For those feeling overwhelmed by the digital clutter, the transition to outdoor activities might seem daunting. Where do you start, and how do you incorporate these activities seamlessly into your daily routine? Start with small steps. Consider integrating brief walks into your daily schedule. A ten-minute walk during a lunch break or after dinner can start to rewire habitual reliance on screens for entertainment and relaxation. Over time, these little breaks can become a cherished part of your daily routine, providing clarity and energy.

Structured outdoor activities can also serve as excellent entry points. Community sports leagues or outdoor fitness classes offer opportunities for engagement while still being organized enough to feel approachable for those new to regular outdoor activity. These settings provide not only physical benefits but are also fantastic opportunities for social interaction, helping to build a sense of community.

It's important to address the balance between organized and free play. While both have their merits, it is the unstructured, child-led play that often reaps the greatest rewards in creativity and personal satisfaction. When children are left to their own devices (not the electronic ones), they learn to develop a love for exploration and discovery. They learn patience as they watch a line of ants or the gentle sway of the trees, and through this, they cultivate an appreciation for the world's natural rhythms.

Encouraging outdoor play requires commitment and creativity from both parents and guardians. Consider converting a part of your backyard into an engaging space with diverse textures and toys that inspire imaginative play. Whether it's a simple sandbox, a few climbing rocks, or a garden area where kids can plant and watch their efforts grow, the aim is to create a diverse and welcoming environment.

Another aspect to consider is the role of outdoor excursions in educational growth. Nature is the perfect classroom. It's one thing to read about ecosystems, but another to experience them firsthand. Local nature trails and reserves can provide children with insights into wildlife, geology, and conservation that a textbook or screen can't offer. These real-life lessons encourage a deeper understanding and respect for our environment.

Incorporating outdoor activities also means setting boundaries with technology. Create tech-free zones or specific times during the day when screens are off-limits, like during family dinners or before bedtime. Communicating these rules clearly and consistently helps set expectations and normalizes the idea that not all fun needs to be achieved through digital means.

It's essential to remember that what works for one family might not suit another. Some might find joy in the simplicity of gardening together, watching the fruits of their labor come to life, while others might thrive on the energy of group sports or the peace found in hiking paths less traveled. The key is to find what excites and intrigues your family, encouraging sustained engagement and enjoyment.

Ultimately, encouraging outdoor play and engagement isn't about restricting technology; it's about expanding the horizons beyond its screen. The goal isn't to eliminate technology from our lives but to carve out moments of peace and presence in an increasingly connected world. Embracing these moments of outdoor engagement can ignite passions, restore balance, and foster a family culture that values both digital and natural worlds.

As families step outside, they reclaim their senses, finding joy not in the artificial glow of a screen but in the vibrant colors of a sunset or the feel of grass beneath their feet. In the end, these are the experiences that cultivate a life rich in presence and connection, helping us all to flourish in harmony with the digital age.

Chapter 14:
Workplace Digital Detox

In today's fast-paced professional environment, where the ping of notifications and the glow of computer screens often set the rhythm of our workdays, finding ways to cultivate focus and tranquility can feel daunting. Yet, the quest for a balanced digital work life is not just possible; it's transformative. Embracing a workplace digital detox isn't about eliminating technology, but rather about redefining how we engage with it, allowing space for deep concentration and meaningful interactions. By establishing intentional boundaries, such as designated tech-free zones or mindful meeting practices, professionals can foster environments that encourage creativity and reduce stress. Whether navigating the demands of a bustling office or the solitude of remote work, learning to manage digital distractions can lead to profound shifts in productivity and well-being. This process is less about restriction and more about empowerment—finding freedom in adaptation and focus. As we redefine our relationship with technology, we open up opportunities for not just career advancement but personal fulfillment and peace.

Promoting Focus in the Office

In today's world, the modern office is a vibrant, interconnected hub buzzing with digital activity. Emails ping, chats interrupt, and notifications nag at your attention, pulling you into a cacophony of endless, fragmented focus. It feels overwhelming at times, doesn't it?

The challenge is clear: How do we promote focus amid this digital whirlwind? Fortunately, there are actionable strategies to carve out a space for concentration and productivity in the office.

Start by reimagining the office environment itself. Before diving into the chaos of an average workday, consider creating dedicated spaces designed solely for focused work. It's about reclaiming physical islands of calm amid the ocean of digital noise. Here's a thought: Why not designate certain areas or rooms in the office as "focus zones" where devices are limited, and interruptions are minimized? Even if spatial constraints exist, promoting a culture where employees appreciate and respect each other's need for quiet time can make a big difference.

This touches on a deeper transformation, one that asks us to rethink our relationship with technology in our professional lives. Embracing principles of digital minimalism within the office can guide individuals to curate what technology really serves their work versus what simply distracts. By identifying which digital tools genuinely enhance productivity, companies can encourage employees to engage more mindfully, using technology as a supportive ally rather than an overbearing presence.

Another piece of the puzzle is cultivating consistent, mindful practices among team members. Regular "mindfulness moments" during the day—time slots when everyone collectively pauses and refocuses—can be surprisingly powerful. These could be short breathing exercises or simple meditations, even just moments to disconnect from screens and connect with the soul. It's about introducing rhythm and breath into what's often a non-stop, high-speed work routine.

It might also be time to revisit policies surrounding digital communication. By evaluating and potentially limiting the times when non-urgent communications can occur, organizations can free employees from the tyranny of the dreaded notification ping. Establishing "communication-free" periods can conserve mental energy and allow employees to immerse themselves fully in their tasks without the perpetual threat of interruption.

Furthermore, the role of leadership in fostering a focus-friendly environment cannot be overstated. Leaders set the tone, and when they model behavior that values deep work and uninterrupted focus, it sends a powerful message. Encouraging leaders to set boundaries, like opting for tech-free meetings when feasible, can gradually shift the office culture towards one that venerates concentration over constant connectivity.

Let's not forget about the tools themselves. In the hands of an intentional user, technology can uplift instead of deplete. Encouraging the use of apps and tools that track time, promote focus, or block distracting sites can enhance the workplace experience. It's about approaching digital tools with the right mindset—one that sees technology as an enabler of productivity rather than a source of distraction.

There's also an openness to embracing analog components in the workday. Physical notepads, whiteboards, and brainstorming sessions uncoupled from digital platforms allow space for unfettered creativity and collaborative thought without digital interruption. Sometimes, hands-on tasks encourage the mind to focus and think critically, free from the digital din.

Of course, promoting focus isn't just an organizational responsibility; it also requires individual commitment. Employees are empowered when they're encouraged to take ownership of their digital habits. Offering training sessions on digital well-being, such as techniques in reducing screen time or the effective use of digital tools, can equip employees with the skills they need to manage distraction effectively.

In the end, promoting focus in the office is about finding balance. It's about harmonizing the demand for connectivity with the human need for undivided attention. As more organizations adopt these practices, they pave the way for a future where the workplace isn't just efficient but also enriched by mindful, meaningful engagement with both the work and the technology that surrounds it.

Navigating Remote Work Challenges

The transition to remote work has been both a blessing and a challenge for many. It offers unprecedented flexibility and the comfort of working from home, but it also comes with unique challenges that can contribute to digital noise and overwhelm. As remote work becomes the norm for many, finding strategies to cope with its challenges is essential for a successful workplace digital detox. By fostering an environment conducive to productivity and mental well-being, we can make remote work a fulfilling and balanced experience.

One of the most significant challenges in remote work is the blurring of boundaries between professional and personal life. When your home becomes your office, it's easy to find yourself checking emails at odd hours or working late into the night. This lack of separation can lead to burnout and stress. Establishing clear work boundaries is crucial. Create a dedicated workspace, and try to stick to regular working hours as much as possible. Communicate these boundaries to others, both at work and at home, to set realistic expectations.

Working remotely often entails increased reliance on technology, making it hard to unplug and disconnect meaningfully. Video conferences, instant messaging, and constant notifications can lead to digital fatigue. To prevent this, make conscious decisions about when to be online and when to take breaks. Schedule regular intervals to step away from screens, allowing eye rest and mental rejuvenation. Just as we respect the need for lunch breaks, technology breaks should also become part of our routine.

Isolation is another challenge many face while working remotely. The lack of face-to-face interactions can lead to feelings of loneliness and disconnection. Building a sense of community, even virtually, is vital. Regularly check in with colleagues through video chats or conference calls that focus on social interaction rather than just work. Join online communities or forums related to your interests to expand your network and maintain a connection with the outside world. It may not fully replace in-person interaction, but sharing ideas and experiences with a supportive group can mitigate loneliness.

The digital tools we rely on can become both assets and distractions. Managing these tools effectively involves setting priorities and using them mindfully. Start by auditing the applications and tools you use daily. Are there apps that clutter your attention or ones that help streamline your workflow? Keep only what enhances productivity and reduces stress. Tools should serve us, not the other way around. Consider implementing techniques like time-blocking or the Pomodoro Technique to maintain focus and minimize distractions.

With remote work, the challenge of self-regulation becomes more apparent. Without the natural cues of an office environment to guide us, it is crucial to foster self-discipline and motivation. Developing a routine can provide structure and a sense of normalcy. Begin your day with a morning ritual that helps transition from personal to professional mode. It could involve exercise, reading, or listening to music—anything that energizes you and sets a positive tone for the day. Similarly, create an evening ritual to signal the day's end, helping to unwind and break from work mode.

Amid these challenges, remember the importance of self-compassion and flexibility. Remote work is an adjustment, and it's okay to have days that feel less productive. Recognize your achievements, regardless of size, and adjust goals if needed. Sometimes, what we need is a pause to recalibrate. When the typical work hours or conditions don't apply, finding what works for you is essential. We're all navigating uncharted waters, and allowing yourself the grace to adapt is part of a healthy remote work life.

Furthermore, harness the advantages of remote work to pursue a more deliberate and intentional digital experience. Use the flexibility to explore new hobbies or interests offline. Whether it's gardening, painting, or learning to cook, these activities can provide a refreshing break from screen time. Embrace analog options during breaks to refocus and recharge. This balance can lead to newfound resilience in both personal and professional spheres.

In navigating remote work challenges, cultivating a mindful approach to technology use is vital. It involves not just maintaining professional responsibilities but also ensuring personal well-being. By setting boundaries, managing tools wisely, and embracing offline activities, we can transform the remote work landscape into one of opportunity—a chance to redefine our relationship with technology and create a healthier, more balanced life.

Chapter 15:
Digital Minimalism for Students

In the digital whirlwind that defines student life today, finding clarity can feel like chasing shadows. The relentless pull of screens often blurs the line between learning and distraction, making digital minimalism a vital strategy for both academic success and personal well-being. By consciously selecting educational tools that enhance rather than hinder focus, students can pave a path to deeper understanding and sustained concentration. It's about striking a balance, where technology serves as a bridge to knowledge, not a barrier. Embracing study techniques that minimize unnecessary screen time allows students to reclaim their attention, fostering an environment where ideas can flourish unimpeded by digital noise. This intentional approach empowers students to harness the benefits of technology while remaining grounded in the present, ultimately crafting a more mindful and fulfilling educational journey.

Study Techniques for Reduced Screen Use

In today's fast-paced digital world, students often find themselves in a tug-of-war with the screens that dominate their lives. From smartphones to tablets and laptops, these devices have become nearly inseparable companions in the academic journey. However, to truly embrace digital minimalism, one must carve out strategies that reduce screen dependence, promoting a healthier, balanced study experience. Through intentional techniques and mindful choices, students can regain control over their study habits, moving closer to a saner relationship with technology.

One of the most effective ways to reduce screen time is through the adoption of analog study methods. More than a nostalgic nod to the past, using paper and pen can help increase information retention and comprehension. Writing notes by hand has been shown to engage cognitive processes differently than typing, encouraging students to process material more deeply. This technique doesn't just enhance learning—it also serves as a meditative break from the glare of screens.

Implementing the Pomodoro Technique can also aid in minimizing screen exposure. This time-management method involves studying in focused bursts of twenty-five minutes followed by short breaks. During these breaks, students can engage in activities away from screens, such as stretching, going for walks, or even doing a quick meditation session. This approach not only helps reduce the overall time spent on devices but also boosts productivity by preventing burnout and maintaining high levels of concentration during study periods.

Creating a dedicated study space is crucial for students aiming to limit their screen use. By establishing an environment specifically designed for concentration, distractions can be better managed. Consider a minimalist desk setup, free of unnecessary electronic devices, to foster focus. Natural lighting and comfortable seating can further enhance this dedicated zone. Encouraging the use of traditional resources, like textbooks or printouts, over online materials can also contribute to minimizing screen time.

Scheduling regular digital detox periods during study sessions can effectively contribute to screen reduction. Students might choose certain hours each day to power down devices entirely, opting instead for reading physical books or solving problems on paper. This conscious unplugging not only aids in visual rest but also allows cognitive bandwidth to reset, leading to increased creativity and improved problem-solving skills.

Engaging in group study sessions without digital gadgets can be another powerful method. By interacting face-to-face and using whiteboards or flip charts to discuss topics, students build collaborative skills and strengthen their understanding of the material. These gatherings provide a welcome respite from virtual collaboration tools, fostering genuine human connection and engagement. Plus, discussing material with peers can offer new insights, deepening comprehension.

Mindful meditation is an invaluable complementary practice for students looking to cut down screen time. Incorporating short meditation sessions into their study routines can enhance focus and help manage the stress that often accompanies academic pursuits. By deliberately stepping away from screens to center their thoughts, students can improve both mental clarity and their capacity for sustained attention, making study sessions more effective.

Journaling is another analog activity that complements study while reducing screen reliance. Reflecting on learning experiences, setting intentions, or even summarizing key concepts can solidify knowledge and boost metacognitive awareness. Through pen and paper, students can explore their thoughts more honestly and with greater depth than they might through digital means, laying a foundation for personal growth and academic achievement.

When it comes to digital resources necessary for education, such as online databases or e-learning platforms, students should aim to use them in a focused manner. By setting specific objectives before logging on and sticking to planned activities, the urge for digital tangents is reduced. The practice of using a precise list of goals serves as a roadmap, limiting the time spent online and maximizing productivity.

Lastly, sleep plays a pivotal role in improving concentration and reducing the need for excessive screen time. Adequate rest rejuvenates the mind, making study hours more efficient. Establishing an evening routine that excludes screens at least an hour before bedtime can improve sleep quality by reducing exposure to blue light, which disrupts sleep cycles. A restful night ensures that students have the mental stamina for demanding study sessions without defaulting to constant digital engagement.

In summary, reducing screen time during study isn't about eschewing technology entirely—it's about finding a healthy balance that prioritizes mental well-being and effective learning. By consciously choosing techniques that foster deep focus and personal connection, students are empowered to thrive academically without the incessant pull of their digital devices. As they implement these strategies, they make strides toward a more fulfilling educational experience, embracing the principles of digital minimalism where it counts the most.

Balancing Educational Tools and Distractions

In an era where screens dominate every facet of student life, maintaining a clear distinction between educational tools and distractions is pivotal. While technology offers unparalleled access to knowledge and learning resources, it also introduces temptations that are just a click away. For students striving for academic success, mastering this balance is crucial for cultivating a productive learning environment.

The first step in distinguishing educational tools from distractions is recognizing the purpose behind the use of each digital resource. For instance, consider the invaluable benefits of online platforms that offer interactive learning experiences and virtual classrooms. These platforms can amplify understanding and engagement far beyond traditional textbooks. However, within the very same devices, social media notifications and entertainment apps compete for attention, making it easy to veer off course.

Understanding how distractions hijack focus is key. When a student attempts to study or complete assignments, even a single distraction can significantly disrupt concentration. Recent studies have shown that it can take several minutes to regain focus after an interruption. Therefore, creating an optimized study environment by minimizing potential distractions is essential. This could mean installing apps designed to block distractions, setting specific study times, or dedicating a space at home solely for learning, free from unneeded interruptions.

Another approach is leveraging technology to enhance focus rather than detract from it. Apps designed for time management, such as the Pomodoro Technique, encourage students to work in focused sprints with regular breaks. Such methods harness technology's ability to organize time effectively while still allowing moments for relaxation and recharging.

Developing self-awareness is a vital skill in maintaining a balance. Students should regularly reflect on their study habits and identify what serves their education and what hinders it. Journaling daily or weekly about the use of technology can provide insights into how study time is spent and what distractions are most pervasive. Over time, this practice aids in reshaping habits toward more meaningful and disciplined technology use.

Encouraging students to set clear boundaries around their use of digital devices is also effective. Scheduling specific times for checking messages or engaging with social media helps direct focus where it is needed most. This discipline not only boosts academic performance but also fosters a sense of autonomy over one's digital life.

Moreover, the integration of *mindfulness* practices can help students become more intentional with their use of technology. By practicing mindfulness, students learn to pay attention to the present moment and recognize when they are veering toward distraction. Simple techniques, such as deep breathing or brief meditation before a study session, can create a mental state of readiness, allowing students to engage more deeply with their educational tasks.

Collaborative learning environments also play a role in balancing educational tools and distractions. Study groups and peer collaborations, facilitated by digital communication tools, can create a structured setting where students support each other in staying on task. This sense of shared accountability makes it easier to avoid distractions while cultivating collective growth and learning.

Ultimately, finding a balance between educational tools and distractions is about honing **discipline and awareness.** By setting firm boundaries, utilizing technology mindfully, and building a community of learning-focused peers, students equip themselves not only for academic achievement but for lifelong skills in managing technology's pervasive influence.

Make learning apps and tools easily accessible, minimizing time spent searching and maximizing time engaged in educational activities.

Regularly review and uninstall apps or block websites that consistently prove to be sources of distraction.

Encourage physical activities or hobbies away from screens to cultivate a sense of balance and avoid digital fatigue.

Finding this balance not only aids in academic success but enriches students' overall quality of life, paving the way for a healthier and more focused future. By taking the reins of their digital lives, students can transform potential distractions into tools of empowerment and knowledge.

Chapter 16:
Transformative Digital Practices

Amid the cacophony of notifications and relentless digital stimuli, embracing transformative digital practices can shift your relationship with technology from overwhelming to enlightening. Imagine the potential of consuming content mindfully, allowing your attention to rest on what truly nourishes your intellect and spirit, rather than succumbing to the lure of endless scrolling. It's about curating your digital environment with the same care you give to a cherished physical space. Concurrently, cultivating a gratitude practice enhances focus by anchoring you to the present moment, fostering a positive mindset that transcends digital noise. This dual approach empowers you to act with intention, forging a path where technology serves as a tool for enrichment, rather than a source of distraction. By adopting these practices, you're not just managing digital life; you're transforming it into a realm of conscious choice and profound presence, paving the way for a more balanced and fulfilling existence.

Mindful Content Consumption

In a world where screens bombard us with endless streams of information, practicing mindful content consumption becomes an essential skill. As we traverse the digital landscape, it's easy to become ensnared by a whirlwind of information that's often more overwhelming than enlightening. Our days are swallowed by a continuous flow of notifications, news feeds, and media, all vying for our attention. But what if we could turn this around? What if we could transform how we engage with digital content to enhance our lives instead of complicating them?

Mindful content consumption invites us to take a step back and evaluate the digital diet we consume daily. This practice isn't about turning away from digital content altogether; rather, it's about reclaiming agency over the choices we make when interacting with our devices. It's about creating a purposeful relationship with content that aligns with our values and contributes positively to our mental and emotional well-being. Imagine cultivating a balanced content diet that nourishes your mind instead of depleting it.

The first step towards mindful content consumption is awareness. Becoming conscious of our habits and emotional responses to what we consume online is crucial. Are there certain types of content that leave you feeling drained or anxious? Are there times when scrolling through social media leaves you with a sense of inadequacy or restlessness? Take note of these instances. Awareness is not just the first step; it sets the stage for change, allowing us to make small, deliberate shifts in our engagement with digital content.

Once aware, it's essential to curate your digital environment thoughtfully. Ask yourself: What voices do I want to invite into my day? What information is truly valuable? Start by cleaning up your feed. Unfollow accounts that offer little value or that perpetuate negativity, and instead follow those that inspire, educate, or bring joy. By intentionally selecting the content you let in, you can ensure your digital interactions are more likely to uplift rather than drain you.

In addition to curating your digital spaces, setting boundaries is key. This means establishing time limits for content consumption and scheduling periods of intentional disconnection. For instance, designate tech-free periods in your day devoted to activities that don't involve screens. These breaks will give your mind the chance to recharge and can enhance your appreciation for the digital content you consume afterwards.

An often overlooked aspect of mindful content consumption is the importance of single-tasking. We live in a multitasking culture, often juggling several pieces of content at once. However, studies consistently show that multitasking is less effective than we think. By focusing on one piece of content at a time, we can engage more deeply and extract more value from it. Consider devoting your full attention to reading a single article or watching a video all the way through, rather than skimming or fast-forwarding. You'll likely find the experience more rewarding.

Furthermore, mindful consumption extends beyond what we're viewing or listening to; it includes the emotional and cognitive load that content imparts. Engaging actively with content instead of passively consuming it can build a more meaningful relationship with the digital world. Reflect on the ideas presented, discuss them with others, and integrate newfound knowledge into your life. By doing so, you're not just consuming content; you're interacting with it, which leads to deeper understanding and retention.

It's also important to recognize the role of positive digital interactions. Building connections with like-minded individuals or joining communities that foster growth and support can transform the way we experience digital spaces. These connections can provide a sense of belonging and purpose in our online interactions, countering the isolating effects of mindless scrolling.

While digital spaces offer a wealth of information and connection, it's crucial to remember that not all content serves our best interests. Practicing skepticism and discernment in evaluating sources and information can protect us from misinformation and cognitive biases. Challenge content that seems dubious and seek multiple perspectives to form a well-rounded understanding of complex issues.

The journey towards mindful content consumption is deeply personal and requires introspection. Reflect on what you consume and why, and reassess regularly. As you refine your practices, acknowledge that perfection isn't the goal; instead, aim for progress and understanding. Our relationship with technology is constantly evolving, and thus, so should our strategies for engaging with it mindfully.

As with most transformative practices, the rewards of mindful content consumption outweigh the effort involved. By fostering a discerning approach to digital content, you create space for growth, balance, and fulfillment. This practice opens the door to a more intentional digital life, allowing you to harness the benefits of technology without being overwhelmed by its noise.

Cultivating a Gratitude Practice

In today's fast-paced digital world, gratitude can seem like a quaint concept, tucked away amidst a swirling tide of notifications and endless scrolling. Yet, it holds a transformative potential to reshape our relationship with technology. Gratitude, when cultivated thoughtfully, can become a powerful anchor, allowing us to stay grounded and appreciate the present, even as digital demands pull at our attention.

Integrating a gratitude practice into our digital lives may seem challenging, but it boils down to small, conscious choices. It's about placing value on moments of appreciation over digital distraction. Imagine starting each day with a simple ritual: writing down three things you're grateful for, be it the warmth of your morning coffee, a message from a loved one, or even the quiet before the world wakes up. This practice doesn't just increase personal awareness; it serves as a reminder of what's genuinely fulfilling in our lives beyond the ephemeral digital buzz.

Research has shown that gratitude improves emotional resilience and enhances overall well-being. In the context of digital overload, it provides a buffer against the stressors of constant connectivity. It helps us to focus on what truly matters, redirecting energy from the pursuit of likes and shares to cultivating meaningful interactions and personal contentment. By nurturing gratitude, we rewire our brains to prioritize depth over breadth, fostering connections that matter rather than superficial digital engagements.

While contemplating the power of gratitude, it's essential to consider how technology can both aid and hinder this practice. On one hand, digital tools and apps offer structured formats for daily gratitude journaling, introducing prompts and reminders at convenient times. On the other, the very devices that facilitate our practice can all too easily become another source of distraction. Maintaining balance is key; the technology should support rather than obscure our journey toward a more appreciative life.

Consider taking advantage of digital platforms to express and share gratitude. Offering thanks via a simple email or an online post can inspire others, creating a ripple effect that extends beyond personal boundaries. Digital gratitude isn't about seeking validation; rather, it's about sharing genuine appreciation, which can enhance our connectedness and mutual understanding in virtual spaces.

Creating boundaries around our tech usage is crucial when cultivating a gratitude practice. Allocating device-free moments—like during meals or walks—allows us to focus more intently on the world and people around us. These pauses offer opportunities to reflect on and absorb the positive aspects of our lives, unfiltered by digital noise. By intentionally stepping back from our screens, we open ourselves to a more mindful experience of gratitude.

Integrating gratitude with digital minimalism can redefine your relationship with technology. By choosing to use technology in a way that enhances life rather than dominates it, gratitude naturally follows. This practice fosters an appreciation for simplicity, teaching us that fulfillment often arises from less rather than more.

Acknowledging the role of gratitude in digital spaces also means recognizing its limitations. While expressing gratitude online can be meaningful, physical or personal expressions often have a more profound impact. A handwritten note or a verbal acknowledgment can convey sincerity and emotional depth in ways digital words sometimes fail to do.

Ultimately, the essence of cultivating gratitude lies in regular practice. Consistency turns gratitude from a momentary thought into a lifestyle. Daily reflections can lead to deeper insights into what we value and cherish. Over time, these insights shape our digital interactions, encouraging us to use technology in ways that reflect our priorities and enhance rather than erode our peace of mind.

Incorporating gratitude into your digital life demands effort and intentionality, but the rewards—clarity, focus, presence—are invaluable. As we navigate a landscape increasingly dictated by digital noise, gratitude provides a counterbalance, offering calm and perspective. It's time to embrace this transformative practice, ensuring our digital experiences are as enriching and meaningful as the lives we aspire to lead.

Chapter 17:
The Power of Unplugging

In a world saturated with constant connectivity, the act of unplugging emerges as a transformative force, offering a sanctuary for the mind and soul. By consciously stepping away from screens, we give ourselves the gift of presence, rediscovering moments of clarity and inner peace amidst the digital clamor. Scheduling regular tech breaks doesn't just momentarily liberate us; it fosters long-term benefits of creativity, mindfulness, and genuine connection with our surroundings. This simple yet powerful practice allows us to recalibrate our priorities and invites spaciousness into our reflections and interactions. Unplugging, although seemingly counterintuitive in a hyper-connected age, does not signify falling behind; instead, it provides a profound opportunity to move forward with intention and authenticity.

Scheduling Regular Tech Breaks

In today's hyper-connected world, where continuous notifications and digital demands are the norm, scheduling regular tech breaks is an essential strategy for maintaining balance and mental well-being. The hustle and bustle of daily life can consume our attention, affecting our ability to focus and truly live in the moment. Regular tech breaks aren't just about pausing the constant stream of emails and messages; they're about reclaiming moments of peace and freedom from the digital noise that often engulfs us.

The need for these breaks stems from the anxiety and fatigue that constant digital engagement can produce. When we're absorbed in technology, it's easy to lose sight of the importance of downtime. However, intentionally scheduling tech breaks creates space for mental clarity and emotional reset. This can lead to reduced stress levels and an overall sense of calm. Moreover, stepping away from screens allows us to reconnect with the physical world, fostering a deeper appreciation for the simple, yet profound experiences around us.

Regular tech breaks are as vital as any other aspect of our well-being routines. Just as we dedicate time to exercise or meditation, incorporating these breaks into our daily schedule can cultivate a healthier relationship with technology. You might start with small intervals, such as ten-minute breaks every hour, gradually extending these periods as you grow more comfortable with the silence. The idea is to create a rhythm that allows your mind to rest and recharge, improving focus and productivity when you do return to your digital tasks.

Consider integrating tech-free activities into your break times. This could be as simple as going for a walk, engaging in a hobby, or practicing mindfulness. The key is to find activities that nourish your soul. For some, this might mean getting lost in a good book; for others, it might be gardening or cooking a meal from scratch. These analog experiences provide a counterbalance to the digital world, offering sensory engagement that screens can't replicate.

Creating a schedule for tech breaks doesn't have to be rigid. Tailor it to your needs and lifestyle. Perhaps begin with an hour away from screens in the morning before your day gains momentum. Use this time to set intentions for the day or simply enjoy a quiet breakfast. In the evening, maybe an hour or two before bedtime could be dedicated to winding down without screens. This not only aids in improving sleep but also allows for reflection and the opportunity to process the day's events without interruptions.

Of course, challenges will arise. Scheduling these breaks might seem daunting in the face of digital obligations. Work demands, social media engagement, and the fear of missing out (FOMO) can make the prospect of stepping away even temporarily feel impossible. However, it's important to remember that you control your schedule, not the digital devices around you. Adjust your mindset to view these breaks as opportunities rather than constraints.

To assist with sticking to your schedule, leverage tools designed to promote digital well-being. Many apps now offer features to help monitor and limit screen time, remind you to take breaks, and even block certain apps during designated hours. These tools act as a bridge, guiding you toward a more mindful relationship with technology and supporting your journey to minimize distractions.

Moreover, sharing your intentions with friends or family can foster a sense of accountability. When others know you're trying to create healthier habits, they're more likely to support you, and you might even inspire them to take their own tech breaks. This can lead to collective digital detox activities, like tech-free dinners or group outings, strengthening your connections offline.

Incorporating regular tech breaks is a pivotal step towards digital minimalism and mindful tech use. It's about consciously choosing when and how to engage with technology, rather than being dictated by it. As you begin to see the benefits of these breaks — from increased focus and creativity to reduced stress and improved relationships — you'll likely find yourself wondering how you ever managed without them.

As the world grows increasingly digital, the art of unplugging becomes ever more crucial. Scheduling regular tech breaks is a powerful tool for fostering this balance, enabling us to lead lives enriched with intention and presence, free from the chains of unrelenting digital distractions. Embracing these breaks wholeheartedly can transform your daily life, providing a much-needed reset and helping you navigate the digital age with grace and mindfulness.

Harnessing the Benefits of Disconnection

In a time when the digital hum surrounds us incessantly, taking a deliberate step back might seem radical. Yet, the rewards of consciously embracing moments of disconnection can be both profound and transformative. In acknowledging the power of unplugging, we don't just sever ties—temporary as they may be—with our devices; we also cultivate a space for insight, creativity, and renewal.

Disconnection is not about rejecting modern technology; rather, it's an act of asserting control over how and when we engage with the digital world. When we deliberately choose to unplug, we allow our minds a much-needed respite. These pauses are crucial in reducing the cognitive load that constant connectivity imposes on us. By scheduling regular intervals free of digital interruptions, we can enhance our mental clarity and boost our productivity once we're back online.

Moreover, stepping away from screens provides an opportunity for self-reflection and introspection, which are often curtailed by our hurried digital lives. During these moments, we can explore our thoughts and emotions with greater clarity, gaining insights into what's truly important. This self-awareness is a crucial component in fostering deeper well-being and aligning our daily actions with our core values.

Beyond personal insight, disconnection presents the chance for richer interpersonal experiences. When we commit to being fully present with those around us, we nurture relationships and foster a sense of community. Imagine a dinner without the distraction of notifications or a conversation that isn't punctuated by the quick glance at a phone. Such moments become rare opportunities to engage deeply and meaningfully with others.

But the benefits aren't solely internal. Studies have shown that intentionally discharging from digital inputs allows our brains to engage with different wavelengths of thought, including daydreaming and creative ideation. By disconnecting, we provide the brain with the freedom to wander, facilitating the piecing together of disparate ideas and inspiration from unexpected sources.

Setting clear boundaries and schedules for disconnection can lead to lasting habits. Whether it's a tech-free morning routine or designated screen-free zones in your home, these practices help in cultivating a lifestyle that prioritizes balance and intention. The boundaries we create remind us that our lives are truly enriched when they're not entirely dictated by screens.

It's also important to recognize that the benefits of disconnection extend to our physical well-being. Taking breaks from devices relieves eyestrain and reduces the risk of ailments associated with prolonged screen time. Similarly, these breaks encourage us to move around more frequently, aiding in overall health and fitness.

While the concept of disconnection might spur anxiety over missing out or falling behind, embracing it gradually can help mitigate these concerns. Starting small with brief retreats from technology can assist us in acclimating to progressive longer periods without digital dependence. Over time, these practices help lay the foundation for a more mindful relationship with technology.

Empowering ourselves with the choice to unplug isn't just about subtraction—it's about gaining the freedom to engage more fully with our offline lives. The act of disconnecting provides a canvas for authentic experiences that are frequently overshadowed by the digital tidal wave. As we harness the benefits of disconnection, we step closer to understanding ourselves, others, and the world around us with greater depth and sincerity.

Finally, remember, the practice of unplugging isn't fixed to rigid standards. It's as unique as the individuals who choose to engage in it. By honing a personal disconnection routine that fits our lifestyle and needs, we unlock the pathway to a more fulfilling life both on and offline.

Chapter 18:
The Influence of Tech Companies

As we navigate the digital landscape, it's crucial to recognize the profound influence tech companies exert over our lives. These entities, with their vast resources and unparalleled reach, shape the technologies that have become integral to our daily routines. Consequently, they wield a significant impact on how we interact with the world and with each other. While their innovations offer convenience and connection, they also encourage behaviors that can lead to distraction and disengagement from the present moment. It's essential to remain mindful of how seamlessly these influences are woven into our habits and to advocate for changes that prioritize our digital well-being. By holding tech companies accountable and pressing for transparent practices, we can work towards a more balanced relationship with technology—one that supports our mental health and enriches our lives, rather than overwhelming them.

Understanding Big Tech's Role

In our quest to live more deliberately in the digital age, it's essential to understand the influence of big tech companies. These titans of technology have woven their presence into nearly every aspect of our lives, shaping behaviors, altering perceptions, and quite literally defining how we connect with each other. Their products and services offer convenience, but they also bring challenges that can disrupt our pursuit of a balanced and fulfilling relationship with technology.

For many, the platforms designed by these companies have become inextricable from daily life. Consider the simple act of communication—once a phone call or face-to-face interaction, now often a stream of messages, emails, or social media updates. Each time we reach for our devices, we're engaging with systems meticulously crafted to capture our attention and, at times, overwhelm our senses. This is no accident; it's a feature of the business models that dominate tech, where the currency is time and attention.

The magnitude and reach of big tech are unprecedented. Companies like Google, Facebook, and Amazon have amassed a level of data about their users that's both impressive and concerning. They analyze this data to predict and even influence user behavior, impacting everything from what news we read to the products we buy. The algorithms that govern their platforms are designed to keep us engaged—sometimes at the cost of our peace and focus.

But it's not just about the algorithms. There's also the design of digital interfaces, which lure us in with bright colors, notifications, and rewards. Have you ever opened an app to check one thing and found yourself scrolling an hour later? You're not alone. The design tactics employed by big tech exploit human psychology, making it increasingly difficult to disconnect. Here, understanding their role is crucial not just for blame assignment but for reclaiming control of our tech use.

In acknowledging big tech's influence, we can't ignore the ethical considerations at play. The responsibility these companies hold extends beyond profits and shareholder value; it involves the well-being of their users. For too long, the emphasis has been on growth and engagement, often at the expense of mental health and privacy. Yet, this recognition also opens the door to advocacy and change.

Individuals and organizations advocate for digital well-being, prompting some companies to take incremental steps toward prioritizing user health. Features that remind us to take breaks, tools for monitoring screen time, and settings for limiting notifications are now common. While these steps are encouraging, it's critical to remember that meaningful change requires constant pressure from informed users demanding accountability and transparency.

Moreover, understanding big tech's role doesn't imply that we must wholly reject their innovations. Rather, it calls for a nuanced approach where we use technology to enhance our lives thoughtfully. Mindful tech use involves harnessing these tools to foster meaningful connections, expand knowledge, and cultivate joy without falling prey to the noise.

Achieving this balance means becoming more selective with our digital engagement. Choosing carefully which platforms to engage with, evaluating how they affect our mood and productivity, and regularly reassessing their place in our lives are vital steps. Engaging in digital minimalism—central to which is minimizing the time spent on these platforms—is itself a form of empowerment.

It's undeniable that the tech landscape will continue to evolve, introducing new features, devices, and challenges. However, by fostering a deeper understanding of big tech's intentions and methods, we empower ourselves to navigate this terrain with intention and clarity. It's about taking back our time, refocusing our attention on what's truly meaningful, and advocating for tech that supports rather than detracts from our well-being.

The journey toward mindful tech use starts with awareness. It calls us to question our habits, understand the forces at play, and strive for a tech life that aligns with our values. As we move forward, recognizing big tech's role is a pivotal part of reimagining our relationship with technology. Armed with this insight, we can make choices that honor our mental space, preserve our focus, and enhance our well-being, creating a digital world that works for us rather than against us.

Advocating for Digital Well-being

In a world where digital technologies have woven themselves into the very fabric of daily life, advocating for digital well-being has never been more critical. The influence of tech companies extends far beyond the gadgets and apps we use; it shapes how we connect, learn, and think. The pressing question is not whether technology is useful—it's how we can manage its impact on our well-being while harnessing its benefits.

Tech companies have a unique position of power and responsibility. They design platforms and products that influence our habits, emotions, and even our mental health. Increasingly, people are recognizing the need to push these corporations to prioritize user well-being in their design. This movement is not about rejecting technology but reshaping its role in our lives. By joining this advocacy, individuals can encourage tech companies to shift towards ethical designs that support mental health and holistic lifestyles.

The design of a product often dictates its usage. Companies can choose to create interfaces that encourage addiction or ones that promote healthy interactions. Advocates for digital well-being argue for the latter, urging tech companies to implement features that limit screen time or promote breaks. Imagine a social media app that rewards you for putting down your phone or a platform that reminds you to take a moment to breathe deeply. Such innovations could transform our relationship with technology, fostering a more balanced digital life.

Furthermore, it's essential for tech companies to increase transparency about how their platforms operate and impact users. This includes sharing data on how algorithms can affect mental health, well-being, and cognitive development. By opening these black boxes, companies can build trust with users and empower them to make informed decisions about their technology use. Users can benefit from choosing digital products that align with their values and goals for well-being.

Advocacy doesn't stop with demanding better design or transparency. It's also about creating a culture where digital well-being is prioritized from the ground up. This requires collaboration among stakeholders, including tech companies, educational institutions, healthcare professionals, and communities. Together, they can develop and promote strategies for integrating digital health literacy into public consciousness.

It's not just the responsibility of tech companies to facilitate digital well-being—individuals must take active roles in demanding these changes. This can be a daunting task, but collective efforts amplify voices, making it easier to drive meaningful change. Joining groups or campaigns focused on digital wellness can provide support and resources to individuals looking to make an impact. When people come together, they can urge tech giants to consider the long-term effects of their products on society.

Beyond pressure from external bodies, there's potential for tech companies to see the value in adopting and championing digital well-being practices. Viewing digital well-being not as an obstacle but as an opportunity to innovate can lead to the development of groundbreaking solutions. This proactive shift may result in healthier human-tech interactions, paving the way for a future where technology acts as a tool for enhancing life rather than hindering it.

The road to achieving widespread digital well-being may be challenging, but its rewards are significant. By fostering environments where both users and creators collaborate on healthy tech ecosystems, everyone can live more mindful, focused, and enriching lives. Advocacy for digital well-being isn't just for those who feel overwhelmed today; it's an investment in a future where digital harmony is the norm.

Individuals overwhelmed by the digital noise can take heart in knowing that change is possible. The path forward involves both personal accountability and collective action—holding tech companies accountable while making intentional choices about technology usage in daily life. By embracing this dual approach, people can reclaim their peace of mind and find meaning beyond the digital waves that often drown it out.

Ultimately, advocating for digital well-being means championing a human-centric view of technology use—one that aligns with intrinsic values and promotes actual human connection. This advocacy focuses on redesigning our digital environments and redefining how technology fits into lives that seek balance, fulfillment, and joy. Together, both individuals and corporations have the power to shape a digital world where everyone thrives.

Chapter 19:
Building a Community of
Intentional Tech Users

Imagine the power of uniting with others who share your desire to redefine tech's role in our lives. That's the essence of building a community of intentional tech users: a space where shared commitment fosters support, inspiration, and collective growth. Everyone's journey to mastering mindful technology use is unique, yet together, we can amplify our efforts and celebrate victories over digital distractions. In these communities, individuals find accountability partners who understand the struggles and triumphs of controlled tech usage. Here, success stories aren't just personal wins but shared triumphs that motivate and guide others along the same path. By nurturing these connections, we create a ripple effect of change, empowering more individuals to reclaim their attention, live purposefully, and breathe a little easier in a world dominated by screens. This collective endeavor not only strengthens our resolve but also builds a movement advocating for a balanced digital life, making it a shared pursuit rather than a solitary struggle.

Finding Support and Accountability

Today, in our constantly connected world, the journey towards intentional technology use can often feel like you're swimming against a strong tide or climbing an uphill path. However, building a community of like-minded individuals can offer both the support and accountability needed to sustain this journey. Finding allies who share your vision and goals can turn your solitary endeavor into a collaborative mission. When individuals come together with a shared purpose, the collective energy and motivation significantly enhance the likelihood of success.

Support can come from various sources. Family and friends are often the first to come to mind, and they can indeed be powerful allies in your quest for balanced tech use. Sharing your goals with them not only provides you with a sounding board but also allows them to help keep you on track. Imagine a household where everyone commits to reducing screen time over family meals. Not only would this make the endeavor more enjoyable, but it would also turn family time into a richer, more engaged experience.

Beyond personal relationships, digital communities have emerged as vital support systems. Online groups dedicated to digital detoxing, minimalism, or mindful technology usage can provide valuable insights and encouragement. These communities are often filled with individuals who have faced similar challenges, offering empathy and practical tips derived from their own experiences. If someone from the group shares a similar struggle and has successfully found a solution, learning from their journey can shorten yours significantly.

That said, accountability plays just as crucial a role as support does. While support offers encouragement and companionship, accountability ensures adherence to commitments and goals. Finding an accountability partner, whether offline or in an online community, can be a game-changer. This person doesn't just cheer you on, but also has the courage and honesty to call you out when you're veering from your goals. They remind you why you embarked on this journey in the first place and help you stay true to your intentions.

The relationship should be reciprocal. Just as your accountability partner supports you, you'll likely take on the same role for them.

Mutual accountability reinforces commitment, as you're less likely to let down someone who's counting on you. Having regularly scheduled check-ins, whether it's weekly phone calls, video chats, or even short messages, can keep both parties aligned with their goals and ensure neither loses sight of their intentions.

Beyond personal accountability, setting communal objectives can also magnify the impact of intentional technology use. For instance, engaging in digital fasting as a group, where each member commits to staying offline during specific times, can dramatically enhance adherence. The shared commitment often acts as a powerful motivator, propelling each participant to remain committed despite potential temptations or distractions.

Furthermore, hosting regular events—be they virtual or physical— that promote digital minimalism can solidify a community's commitment to this lifestyle. Book clubs focusing on pertinent literature, group hikes, or workshops on mindfulness practices can deepen members' investment in this journey. Such events serve as reminders of the collective goals, reinforcing values and strategies in a communal, supportive setting.

In building a community focused on intentional tech use, it's essential to cultivate an environment where sharing is encouraged. Members should feel safe to express their challenges, setbacks, and victories. Celebrating milestones, however small, can build momentum and inspire others to remain steadfast. Similarly, discussing struggles can offer insights, as others may have faced similar challenges and found ways to overcome them.

While online interactions have undeniable value, supplementing digital connections with face-to-face engagements can fortify these relationships. Whenever possible, meeting in person, even if occasional, can deepen connections beyond what digital means can achieve. It further emphasizes the goal of redirecting our focus from screens to real, tangible interactions.

Equally important is the recognition that each individual's journey will be unique. What works well for one person might not be suitable for another. Therefore, the community should emphasize flexibility and adaptability, allowing members to choose pathways that resonate best with their personal lives and goals. Whether it's through group activities, setting personal challenges, or sharing resources, the focus should always remain on empowering each individual to discover and walk their own path.

Investing in the creation and maintenance of these supportive environments fosters a collective resilience. In today's ever-changing digital landscape, having a steadfast community can shield individuals from the fleeting trends and pressures of the broader digital world. It reaffirms the importance of intentional living in a society often consumed by the race towards more, faster, and newer.

Looking to the future, such communities can potentially spark broader societal changes. As more people witness the benefits and spread the principles of mindful technology use, these ideas could ripple outward, influencing wider circles and eventually cultural norms. Each action, no matter how small, contributes to a significant collective impact.

In essence, the spectrum of support and accountability ranges far and wide—from friends to strangers, from digital platforms to in-person gatherings. It's about creating a network that sustains and propels us forward, allowing us to navigate the vast digital landscape with clarity and intention. Together, as a community, we can collectively reclaim our time, attention, and ultimately, our lives. While technology offers us incredible tools, it's how we choose to wield them that defines our experience. With the backing of a community, we are not just users of technology but can become conscious architects of our digital realities.

Sharing Success Stories

In the journey toward becoming intentional tech users, sharing success stories serves as a powerful catalyst. Stories are the threads that weave us together, creating a tapestry of shared experiences and insights. When we exchange narratives of transformation, we do more than just inspire; we foster a sense of community and mutual understanding. We begin to recognize that we aren't alone, and that technology doesn't have to dominate our lives.

Consider the story of Emma, a young professional who found herself drowning in the endless stream of notifications and emails. Every day felt like a battle against distraction, fighting to stay afloat in a sea of digital chaos. Emma knew she needed to make a change, but the prospect of disconnecting seemed daunting. One evening, fueled by a growing desire for peace, she made a commitment to turn her phone off two hours before bed. What started as a small step blossomed into a nightly ritual. She filled her evening hours with reading, meditation, and simply being present. Emma's story is a testament to the power of small intentional changes and the profound impact they can have on our mental well-being.

Another inspiring tale is that of Javier, a college student who felt enslaved by his devices. Social media was a constant lure away from his studies, and his grades were slipping. One day, he stumbled across a digital minimalism workshop on campus. Intrigued, he attended and learned about the impact of device usage on his attention span. He decided to experiment with deleting social media apps from his phone for a week. That week turned into a month, and by the end of the semester, Javier found himself more focused and less anxious. Despite initial fears of missing out, he discovered that the connections he truly valued remained unbroken; they simply shifted to more meaningful interactions offline.

Stories like Emma's and Javier's highlight the empowering nature of taking control over technology. They are reminders that we have the capacity to redefine our relationship with the digital world. By listening to these stories and sharing our own, we build a network of support and accountability. This community becomes a refuge—an oasis in the desert of digital overload.

We also have the tale of an unexpected advocate for digital balance: a small business owner named Carla. As the owner of a boutique bakery, she found herself constantly available via email and social media, struggling to maintain a boundary between her work and personal life. It wasn't until a personal health scare that Carla reevaluated her digital habits. She began setting boundaries by designating "tech-free" times during her day, allowing her to focus on the art of baking and the joy it brings. The transformation led her not only to increased productivity but also to a deeper connection with her customers and employees.

These success stories emphasize perseverance and resilience. They show us that shifting away from digital dependency requires courage and commitment. It may not always be easy, and there'll be setbacks along the way, but each story is a beacon of hope, showing that a more intentional relationship with technology is indeed possible.

It is crucial to recognize that success doesn't mean the same thing to everyone. For some, success may look like reduced screen time and improved mental health; for others, it could mean increased productivity or simply reclaiming time for hobbies and family. The beauty of these stories lies in their diversity. They remind us that our paths toward digital balance are unique, shaped by our individual needs and values.

How, then, can we effectively share these stories within our communities? Technology, ironically, plays a vital role here. Online forums, social media groups, and community meetings dedicated to digital mindfulness can be excellent platforms for sharing and learning. These spaces provide an opportunity to connect with people from different backgrounds, fostering empathy and understanding. They enable us to witness a multitude of experiences, enriching our own approaches to digital wellbeing.

As we gather and share these tales, let's not forget the importance of celebrating our progress—no matter how small. Recognition of these achievements not only motivates the storyteller but also inspires others to embark on their journeys. Whether through blog posts, podcasts, or a simple diary entry, documenting these stories can offer valuable insights and lessons for others who might be struggling with similar challenges.

Moreover, sharing success stories can drive wider societal change. When we collectively voice our experiences and solutions, we create a groundswell of demand for healthier tech practices. This can influence policy changes within workplaces or educational institutions, prompting a shift toward environments that prioritize digital wellness over constant connectivity.

In the end, these stories remind us that we are not powerless against the behemoth of technology. Together, we can forge a path toward a more balanced digital life. Each story shared is a step toward reclaiming our time, our focus, and ultimately, our peace.

Let's continue to tell these stories, creating an ever-expanding archive of successes that will guide us and future generations towards intentional tech use. After all, our collective wisdom is one of the greatest tools we have in the quest for balance and mindfulness in the digital age.

Chapter 20:
Technology and Sleep

A restful night's sleep feels like a distant dream when screens dominate our evenings. Our affinity for the hypnotic glow of technology often sneaks into the sanctuary of sleep, where it wrestles with our circadian rhythms, disrupting the harmony we yearn for. Yet, understanding this interplay empowers us to reclaim control. We can become allies of our slumber by creating environments conducive to rest—spaces where blue light is banished and tranquility rules. This is more than just a bedtime routine shift; it's an act of self-compassion. By consciously managing tech use as dusk falls, we gift ourselves the serenity of a truly restful night and pave the way for rejuvenation. In doing so, we don't just transform our evenings, we transform our lives, reinforcing a sustainable and peaceful balance between rest and activity.

Establishing a Sleep-Friendly Environment

In today's hyper-connected world, the seamless integration of technology into nearly every aspect of our lives can often seem indispensable. Yet, this constant digital immersion can significantly disrupt one of the most essential aspects of our well-being: sleep. Creating a sleep-friendly environment is more vital than ever to ensure that our interactions with technology don't undermine our rest. By intentionally crafting an environment conducive to sleep, we reclaim our nights for what they were meant to be—a time for rest, recovery, and renewal.

Understanding the science of sleep can empower you to make informed decisions about your pre-bedtime technology use. Sleep isn't just about closing your eyes and drifting off; it's a series of complex cycles that play a critical role in cognitive processing, emotional regulation, and physical repair. When technology disrupts these cycles, the consequences ripple through every aspect of our lives, affecting everything from mood and productivity to our health.

Creating a sleep-friendly environment starts with examining the physical space where you rest. Start by evaluating your bedroom through a lens of comfort and tranquility. Is it cluttered with gadgets or glowing with blinking lights? If so, these elements could be interfering with your ability to fall and stay asleep. The ideal sleep environment is one where technology is minimized—an oasis from your bustling digital life. Consider the bedroom as a sanctuary, a place where simplicity reigns and distractions are limited.

Lighting plays a crucial role in signaling to your body that it's time to wind down. Our natural sleep-wake cycles are largely influenced by light exposure, a fact increasingly underappreciated in our artificially lit and screen-dominated environments. Dimming the lights as you approach bedtime can mimic the setting sun, nudging your body towards relaxation. Warm, ambient lighting can compensate for the harshness of backlit screens, allowing your brain to produce the melatonin needed to signal sleep readiness.

Some simple changes can make a big impact, such as investing in blackout curtains and ensuring that all electronic devices emit no light while idle. Devices can also produce distracting noise. Therefore, establish quietude by relocating any items that buzz, ping, or hum to another room. These small adjustments can help cultivate a tranquil environment to slip effortlessly into slumber.

On the list of nocturnal interferences, the use of electronics at night typically ranks high. The blue light emitted from phones, tablets, and laptops is notorious for its ability to suppress melatonin, yet many of us reach for our devices out of habit or the desire to unwind at the end of a long day. To mitigate this, consider adopting tech-free routines before bed. Engaging in activities that promote relaxation, such as reading a paperback or practicing gentle stretching, can ease the transition from wakefulness to rest.

Routine is a powerful ally in establishing a sleep-friendly environment. Human bodies thrive on regular schedules, and having a habitual bedtime ritual can make a substantial difference in sleep quality. Think of these routines as a series of gentle cues telling your brain that it's time to disengage from the rigors of day-to-day life and prepare for rest. Whether it's sipping herbal tea, listening to calming music, or jotting down thoughts in a journal, consistent practices can anchor your nighttime state of mind.

Mindfulness also finds its place in the sleep environment. Incorporating mindfulness techniques into your evening routine can shift focus away from digital stimulation and towards an internal state of calmness. Techniques such as focused breathing or progressive muscle relaxation can slow racing thoughts and ease the tension that often accompanies the transition to bed. These mindful moments allow us to embrace stillness and let go of the incessant urge to keep checking notifications or emails.

If the allure of technology proves too strong, consider implementing tech-specific strategies to curtail its impact. Many devices and apps have functionalities designed to aid sleep hygiene. Setting your phone to 'Do Not Disturb' mode, instituting app timers, or using software that filters blue light in the evenings can all serve as barriers against tech-induced sleep disruption.

Remember, designing a sleep-friendly environment isn't just about what you remove, but also about what you invite in. The sensory aspects of sound, smell, and touch can enhance your quality of sleep. White noise machines, essential oil diffusers, and high-quality bedding may all contribute to a cozy cocoon that embraces tranquility. These elements foster a holistic atmosphere where serenity is prioritized over sensory overload.

Ultimately, establishing a sleep-friendly environment requires intentionality and a commitment to aligning your practices with the natural rhythms of rest. It's a statement of self-care, recognizing that in a world where technology serves as both a tool and a temptation, reclaiming your sleep is essential to a balanced and fulfilled life.

The path to a restful night might take some finding, but the journey is undeniably worth it. The promise of restorative sleep beckons, inviting you to a place where mind and body are refreshed. Each small choice you make ripples out, creating a bedtime space that honors a peaceful disconnect, ushering you into the gentle embrace of night.

The Impact of Blue Light

The pervasive glow of screens has silently seeped into our daily routines, often without us realizing its profound impact on our sleep patterns. In our quest for constant connectivity, many of us have not considered the effects of blue light emanating from these devices. While the transition to a digital-first world presents numerous benefits, it's crucial to understand how this invisible light may be disrupting one of our most essential human needs: sleep.

Blue light, extensively emitted by smartphones, tablets, computers, and LED lights, mimics the brightness of daylight. This simulation can trick our brains into believing it's still daytime, thereby interfering with our circadian rhythms. Melatonin, the hormone responsible for signaling our bodies to wind down and prepare for rest, becomes suppressed. When our melatonin levels are disrupted, the delicate balance governing sleep and wake cycles is thrown into disarray, leading to difficulty falling or staying asleep.

In a world where digital noise inundates our senses, understanding the unintended consequences of blue light exposure can empower us to reclaim restful nights. As we engage with digital devices late into the night, we inadvertently sacrifice not just sleep quantity but quality. This artificial illumination skews our body clocks, leaving us feeling weary and cranky come morning. To achieve a fulfilling relationship with technology, it's imperative to strike a balance that doesn't undermine our need for restorative sleep.

Consider the allure of the digital glow, often inviting us to scroll endlessly through social feeds or binge-watch another episode, especially when we face stress or anxiety. These habits breed habitual exposure to blue light, eroding the sacred boundary between our waking and sleeping lives. Redressing this imbalance isn't about abandoning technology altogether but about adopting mindful practices that prioritize our well-being over mindless consumption.

Chronic exposure to blue light before bedtime can exacerbate the cycle of digital overwhelm, contributing to a relentless sense of fatigue. This fatigue does not merely reflect in sluggish mornings but affects cognitive functions, mood stability, and overall health. Disturbed sleep can compound feelings of anxiety and depression; hence, addressing blue light exposure is also crucial for mental well-being, as explored earlier in discussions about technology's impact on mental health.

Creating an intentional environment that encourages restful sleep involves regulating blue light exposure. Technologies such as blue light filters on devices, applications enabling warmer tones during night-time browsing, and blue light-blocking eyewear offer practical solutions to mitigate these effects. However, these technological aids should complement, not replace, healthier bedtime routines that limit screen time.

Imagine your bedroom as a sanctuary from the day's digital demands. Establishing a screen-free zone before sleep can be transformative, steering our nightly rituals towards analog pursuits. Simple acts like reading a book, practicing mindfulness exercises, or engaging in calming hobbies radiate a soothing impact, enhancing sleep quality by allowing natural melatonin production to occur uninhibited.

Moreover, advocating for digital downtime aligns seamlessly with the principle of fostering meaningful and intentional interactions with technology. By consciously deciding when and how we expose ourselves to blue light, we nurture a cycle of positive habits that extend beyond the night and into brighter, more focused days. In balancing our embrace of digital convenience with respect for our biological needs, we become more receptive to life beyond the screen.

It's all about choices—a deliberate shift to leave behind the clutches of digital overload when the day winds down. This shift becomes not just a practice but a philosophy, where technology serves rather than dictates our lives. In this dance of light and dark, we hold the power to choreograph a harmony between our digital and physical worlds, where restful sleep amplifies our everyday potential.

Reflect on how a clear mind, nurtured by unbroken rest, fuels creativity, bolsters emotional resilience, and enhances productivity. As blue light dims and fades, its metaphorical shadows recede, allowing our true selves to emerge with renewed vigor and clarity. Yet, this transformation doesn't occur in isolation but as part of a broader journey toward being intentional with our technology use. Together, these efforts create the foundation for a life that embraces balance, focus, and enduring peace.

Chapter 21:
Cultivating Presence in the Digital Age

In a world that never seems to sleep, where notifications and alerts demand our constant attention, cultivating presence becomes both a challenge and necessity. More than ever, it's crucial to anchor ourselves in the moment amidst the cacophony of the digital age. When we're mindful, we reclaim the power to steer our focus, immersing ourselves fully in whatever task, conversation, or reflection we're engaged in. Practicing mindful breathing, a technique that can be as simple as a few deep breaths, allows us to reset and ground, cutting through the haze of digital chatter. As we engage fully in each moment, with intent and purpose, we nurture a sense of calm and fulfillment. This presence transcends screens and gadgets, fostering connections with ourselves and those around us. It's about being here, now, and allowing that presence to guide how we interact with technology—not as a distraction but as a tool for meaningful engagement. The road to a mindful relationship with technology is paved with intention and practice, enabling us to enrich our lives with depth and presence, instead of drifting through a digital cloud. Embracing this mindfulness, we find a harmony that nurtures our well-being, helping us to carve out moments of tranquility amid the digital rush.

Practicing Mindful Breathing

In a world vibrating with the incessant hum of devices, notifications, and digital demands, the simplicity of a deep breath offers a gentle refuge. It's an invitation to step away from the constant pull of technology and anchor ourselves in the present moment. Mindful breathing is more than just an act of respiration; it's a pivotal skill helping to cultivate presence amid digital chaos. By paying close attention to each inhalation and exhalation, we begin to create a buffer between ourselves and the storm of digital noise.

Practicing mindful breathing can be your compass to navigate the overwhelming digital landscape. Begin by finding a quiet space, free from digital distractions. This can be a corner in your home or a spot in nature where the sounds of the real world overshadow the clatter of the virtual one. Sitting comfortably, allow your hands to rest on your knees or lap. Close your eyes and focus on your breath. Feel the cool air as it enters your nostrils and the warmth as it leaves. Imagine each breath as a gentle wave, soothing and constant.

Breathing mindfully doesn't demand hours of your time. Start with just five minutes a day, gradually increasing as you become more comfortable. The beauty of this practice is its portability; whether you're at your desk, in a meeting, or waiting for your coffee to brew, a few mindful breaths can be transformative. It acts as a reset button, offering clarity and calm in moments of digital overwhelm. Over time, this practice not only enhances your focus but also enriches your interactions with technology, making them more intentional and less reactive.

Scientific studies underscore the effectiveness of mindful breathing. Research indicates that focused, deep breathing can lower cortisol levels—the body's stress hormone. This practice reduces anxiety, enhances concentration, and aids in better decision-making, countering the effects of digital fatigue. Moreover, as you toggle between tasks and notifications, mindful breathing reestablishes your control over attention, steering it away from the distractions that technology often imposes upon you.

Let's explore a simple technique known as "box breathing," which is especially useful when digital demands feel overwhelming. Imagine tracing a square in your mind: inhale for a count of four, hold for a count of four, exhale for four, and pause again for four. Repeating this cycle helps regulate your heartbeat, making it easier to manage stress. This method is favored by everyone from Navy SEALs to high-performing executives. It's a testament to how something so simple can wield immense power in maintaining mental equilibrium.

Mindful breathing is not just an individual practice but a communal one, too. Consider incorporating it into digital meetings or family time. As meetings start, taking a collective minute for deep breathing can set a calm tone, encouraging focused discussion rather than scattered thinking. In family settings, mindful breathing can slow down the fast pace of everyday life, creating pause and presence, fostering deeper connections free from digital interference.

As you continue your journey in cultivating presence, remember that mindful breathing is a skill cultivated with patience and practice. It's not just about breathing but about breathing with intention in the service of greater awareness. Like sharpening a tool, each practice hones your capacity to engage fully, standing as a resilient force against the often relentless nature of digital life. It becomes a ritual of renewal, replenishing your mental energy and redefining your interactions with technology.

For many, the allure of constant connectivity is difficult to resist. The digital world's rapid pace offers frequent rewards of instant gratification, but mindful breathing invites you to experience a different type of fulfillment—one that nurtures well-being and sustenance. It's less about the quick fix and more about the lasting impact that mindful presence can provide. The simple act of breathing can unlock gateways of peace, offering a new perspective that celebrates the present moment over digital distractions.

Integrating mindful breathing into your routine grounds your existence amidst digital chaos. As you inhale deeply and exhale fully, you're not just exchanging oxygen for carbon dioxide; you're reclaiming control over your digital experience. This shift in awareness is pivotal in developing a balanced and fulfilled digital relationship. So, welcome each breath as a faithful companion in your quest for digital clarity and mental tranquility, empowering you to navigate the digital age with purposeful intent.

Engaging Fully in the Moment

In a world where our attention is constantly divided, engaging fully in the moment may seem like an elusive goal. The digital age brings with it an unparalleled level of connectivity, offering information and entertainment at our fingertips. But along with these conveniences comes the ever-present temptation to dip into bits of this and bytes of that, rarely giving anything our complete focus. Yet, the true essence of living—what makes life vibrant and meaningful—often lies in the quality of our presence in each moment.

Engaging fully in the moment isn't just a concept or a catchy slogan; it's a practice that can redefine how we interact with the world around us. It entails a conscious decision to focus attention on the present, to be aware of our surroundings, and to immerse ourselves wholeheartedly in whatever we're doing. Whether it's enjoying a meal, listening to a friend, or simply savoring a quiet moment, being present enhances the experience, nurturing deeper connections and fostering a sense of fulfillment.

There's growing evidence in psychological studies that practicing mindfulness—being present—is a key component of mental well-being. Mindfulness has been shown to reduce stress, improve emotional health, and increase resilience. When we engage fully in the moment, we allow ourselves the space to process experiences more deeply and appreciate them more fully. This kind of engagement doesn't eliminate the challenges we face, but it provides a clearer and calmer perspective to navigate them.

The first step to engaging fully in any moment is acknowledging the mental chatter that usually accompanies us throughout the day. Our minds are experts at running commentary and replays of past events or rehearsing future scenarios. This tendency to drift into the past or future robs us of the ability to savor the very moment we're in. Recognizing this habit is crucial; it's the doorway to cultivating presence.

Consider simple practices that anchor your attention. Start with your breath—arguably the most accessible tool we have. Just a few mindful breaths can bring our focus back to the present and settle a restless mind. Observe each inhalation and exhalation, feeling the rise and fall of your chest. This practice isn't about clearing the mind but about bringing the wandering attention back to the rhythm of breathing, effectively resetting the mental turbulence.

Now, think about your daily routines. How often do you go through them on autopilot, barely noticing the details of the world around you? A mindful approach to these routines can transform mundane tasks into moments of peace and meditation. Whether it's the feel of water during a morning shower or the act of eating a meal, these moments, when experienced fully, become gifts of richness and depth.

A tangible way to connect deeply with the moment is through the practice of single-tasking, an intentional departure from the multitasking that technology often demands. Focus on doing one thing at a time and doing it well. This approach isn't only about optimizing productivity—it's about fostering a state of flow. When in flow, activities are performed with a sense of effortlessness and joy, leading to greater satisfaction and completion.

Connection with others also benefits significantly from presence. Having a conversation without distractions—like the constant ping of notifications—creates space for authentic communication and understanding. It allows us to be attuned to non-verbal cues and the emotional nuances that are otherwise missed. When we listen with empathy and respond thoughtfully, we deepen relationships, building trust and intimacy.

But what about the digital tools that form such an intrinsic part of modern life? They're not going anywhere, nor should they. The objective isn't to reject technology but to integrate it meaningfully. Being mindful about how we use our devices and regulating our interaction with them can help preserve moments for true engagement. Set conscious parameters for device use, such as tech-free dinners or a digital sunset routine—an hour before bed devoid of screens. These boundaries act as a sanctuary for presence.

Moreover, leveraging technology itself can aid in fostering presence. There are numerous applications and tools designed to encourage mindfulness, offering guided meditations, reminders to reflect, or tracks to facilitate focused work periods. They act as bridges between the conveniences of technology and the depth of being fully present. They're simple yet effective ways to incorporate intention into a digitally dense lifestyle.

Engagement, at its core, comes down to intention and choice. We must choose to disrupt the patterns that pull us away from the moment and establish new routines that anchor us within it. This journey requires a compassionate curiosity about our habits and a willingness to make incremental shifts. It's important to remember that you don't have to get it perfect; striving for mindful presence is a lifelong practice, one imbued with progress, patience, and self-compassion.

So, engage with today. Be there fully, knowing that such engagement forms a mosaic of invaluable memories and experiences. Celebrate the small victories, the fleeting vistas glimpsed through dedication to presence. In each one, you may find a renewed sense of clarity and purpose that underpins the chaos of a connected world.

Chapter 22:
Digital Detox Retreats and Challenges

In our hyper-connected world, where the pings and notifications never seem to cease, seeking respite can feel like an act of rebellion. Digital detox retreats and personal challenges are emerging as powerful allies in the quest to reclaim focus and serenity. Imagine stepping into a realm where nature's symphony replaces the constant buzz of technology, offering a sanctuary for the mind and soul. These retreats are not merely about escaping; they're about confronting our reliance on screens to rediscover joy in the present. Structured personal challenges, whether it's a weekend without Wi-Fi or a sunset sans screens, invite us to test the waters of disconnection and to savor the calm that follows. By intentionally carving out tech-free moments, either in guided retreats or personal endeavors, we gain the tools to harmonize our digital and analog lives, nurturing a profound sense of peace and presence.

Benefits of Disconnecting in Nature

In our hyper-connected world, the thought of escaping into the heart of nature can feel like a luxury, maybe even a distant dream. But what if this dream holds the key to unlocking a more balanced relationship with technology? While a digital detox in nature might sound like a retreat from the relentless pace of modern life, it's actually an invitation to reconnect with something far more profound—ourselves and the environment that nurtures us.

Nature has a way of drawing us in with its serene landscapes and calming rhythms. It's in these untouched settings that we begin to understand the restorative power of the great outdoors. Studies have shown that spending time in nature reduces stress, lowers blood pressure, and boosts mood. When we're not distracted by constant notifications and the pull of a digital world, we become fully present. And in that presence, we find peace. It's a peace that's not about escaping life but about experiencing it more fully.

Imagine waking up with the sun, surrounded by the gentle rustle of leaves and the chirping of birds. Gone are the persistent buzzing of your smartphone and the blinding blue glow of screens. Instead, you engage your senses in the world around you. You become aware of the earthy scents of the forest, the vibrant colors of wildflowers, and the symphony of nature's unedited soundtrack. It's a sensory feast that feels increasingly rare in our digital age, yet it offers a wealth of benefits that extend beyond mere relaxation.

Disconnecting in nature also allows us to recalibrate our sense of time. Unlike the relentless rush of daily schedules, nature encourages us to adopt a slower, more mindful pace. There's no urgency to scroll or swipe here. Instead, we realize that time isn't something to be filled or conquered, but rather, something to savor. Engaging with nature helps ground us in the present moment, reminding us that life's richness is found not in doing more, but in experiencing what's around us—and within us.

Moreover, nature has a remarkable capacity for teaching us lessons in simplicity, resilience, and interconnectedness. The intricate balance of an ecosystem can inspire us to reevaluate how we manage our own lives, especially our relationship with technology. Just as each element in nature has its role, we can find our own balance by prioritizing what truly matters. Nature becomes our guide, offering insights into sustainable practices that can be applied to digital minimalism, fostering a genuine appreciation for less.

The benefits extend to enhancing our creative and cognitive capabilities. Without the barrage of digital information, our minds have the space to wander and explore ideas anew. Creative breakthroughs often occur when we're least focused on producing them. A quiet walk through a forest or an unhurried sit by a lake can spark inspiration, as our brains enter a state of restful alertness. This is where innovation thrives, where new perspectives are gained, and where solutions to our tech-induced dilemmas often emerge.

Beyond the individual advantages, disconnecting in nature strengthens our social bonds. Gatherings without digital distractions encourage meaningful conversations and shared experiences, building deeper connections with family, friends, or even ourselves. Outdoor activities promote teamwork, empathy, and a sense of community, counteracting the loneliness that technology can sometimes exacerbate. In nature, we find common ground—where stories are shared, laughter echoes, and memories are created, heartening our spirits.

It's crucial to acknowledge that a retreat into nature might not be feasible for everyone all the time. However, integrating nature into our lives, even in small ways, can trigger significant improvements. This could mean a short escape to a local park, tending to a garden, or simply opening a window to let in fresh air and sunlight. The essence of disconnecting is to embrace whatever form connection with nature takes, no matter how modest.

In a nutshell, the act of disconnecting in nature is a journey towards reconnection with ourselves. It nurtures our mental and physical well-being, cultivates presence, enhances creativity, and reinforces community ties. By choosing to unplug and step into the wild, we gift ourselves with clarity and joy that digital interactions rarely offer. It's a transformation that unfolds without fanfare—quietly but profoundly—and it holds the potential to reshape not just how we interact with technology, but how we live our lives.

Structuring Personal Detox Challenges

Digital detox challenges can be transformative for individuals seeking to embrace a healthier relationship with technology. Designing your own personal detox can be an empowering experience, allowing you to tailor the challenge to fit your unique lifestyle and goals. It's essential to approach this process with intentionality, clarity, and self-compassion. By recognizing your digital habits and setting achievable targets, you can create a framework that encourages meaningful change without overwhelming yourself.

Starting with a clear intention is crucial. Reflect on the aspects of digital life you feel are causing disruption or distress. Maybe it's the endless scrolling at night that eats into your sleep or the constant checking of emails that intrudes on your personal time. Once you pinpoint these areas, you can craft specific goals for your detox. These goals should be SMART: Specific, Measurable, Achievable, Relevant, and Time-bound. Perhaps you want to limit social media to one hour a day or designate tech-free zones at home.

Another key component is to outline the parameters of your detox. This means deciding which devices or apps you'll include in the challenge and how you'll limit their use. It's not about cutting out technology completely but creating intentional boundaries that promote well-being. For instance, you might decide that work emails are off-limits after 7 PM or that weekends are reserved for offline activities. These boundaries serve as a gentle reminder that you control how and when technology enters your life.

Next, consider incorporating rituals that reinforce your commitment to the detox. Establishing morning and evening routines that are tech-free can anchor your day in mindfulness and presence. In the morning, you could replace smartphone alarms with a gentle wake-up light, allowing yourself a moment of peace before reaching for technology. At night, perhaps a few minutes of journaling or reading could serve as a calming ritual, signaling the end of digital engagement.

As you embark on this challenge, surround yourself with a supportive environment. Share your intentions with friends or family, explaining the reasons behind your digital detox. Their understanding and encouragement can provide the motivation you need to stick to your goals, and engaging them might inspire similar initiatives in their lives. If you feel comfortable, look for online communities or forums where others share their experiences and challenges, creating a network of accountability and shared aspirations.

Acknowledging your progress is vital. Regularly reflect on your journey, noting changes in your mood, energy, and focus. Are you feeling more present in conversations, or have your stress levels decreased? Celebrate these victories, no matter how small. They signify a shift towards a healthier balance with technology and reinforce the positive impact of the detox. These reflections can also guide you in refining your challenge, making adjustments that align more closely with your evolving needs.

Moreover, balance and flexibility should be fundamental principles during this period. While it's important to be disciplined, it's also crucial to be kind to yourself if setbacks occur. Life's unpredictable nature means there might be days when sticking to your detox feels impossible. That's okay. Allow yourself some grace, using these moments as opportunities to learn rather than self-criticize. Remember, the goal of a digital detox is not perfection but progress and growth.

Finally, as your challenge comes to a close, consider how the insights gained can be integrated into your life moving forward.

Perhaps you've uncovered a newfound love for morning walks or realized that family dinners are more enjoyable without phones. These discoveries can be woven into your daily routine, sustaining the benefits of the detox long-term. It's about creating a digital life that supports your values and aspirations, one that enables you to thrive rather than just survive in today's fast-paced world.

In summary, structuring a personal digital detox challenge requires intentionality, clarity, and compassion. By setting concrete goals, establishing boundaries, and creating supportive rituals, you can navigate technology with greater awareness and purpose. Embrace the journey, remain flexible, and celebrate your progress. The rewards—a more focused, peaceful, and balanced life—are well worth the effort.

Chapter 23:
Leveraging Technology for Good

In a world teeming with digital distractions, leveraging technology for good can feel like finding an oasis in a desert. It's about discovering tools and practices that align with our goals for greater focus and inner peace. Mindfulness apps serve as personal guides, gently nudging us toward moments of calm amidst the chaos. Productivity tools can streamline tasks, freeing up our mental bandwidth for creative and fulfilling endeavors. By conscientiously choosing and using technology, we shift the narrative from overwhelming noise to empowering resources. This shift isn't about rejecting the digital; it's about cultivating a more mindful and intentional relationship with it, transforming technology from a source of stress into a catalyst for personal growth and well-being. Let's embrace the power of technology to enhance our lives, realizing its potential not just for efficiency but also for cultivating meaningful experiences and connections.

Apps for Mindfulness and Focus

In an era dominated by endless notifications and digital noise, finding moments of peace can seem almost impossible. Yet, with thoughtful use of technology, this peace is within reach. Apps designed for mindfulness and focus offer a bridge to reclaiming our mental space amid the chaos. They guide us to not only harness technology's power for good but also to foster a deeper, more intentional connection with our daily lives.

These apps are beneficial not just for those already practicing mindfulness but also for anyone looking to break free from the frantic pace of modern digital life. Mindfulness apps often include features like guided meditations, breathing exercises, and daily reminders to pause—tools that are vital for nurturing a calm mind in an ever-expanding sea of information. For many, integrating these practices into daily routines can be life-changing, providing a structured path to regain focus and mental clarity.

Consider apps like Headspace and Calm, which offer structured programs that help users begin and maintain a mindfulness practice. They provide guided meditations led by experienced instructors, ranging from just a few minutes to deeper, more extensive sessions. These sessions allow individuals to develop a practice that fits their schedule and needs, which is crucial for creating a sustainable habit.

For those aiming for better focus, apps like Forest and Focus@Will offer innovative approaches. Forest rewards users for staying off their devices by growing a virtual tree that flourishes only with uninterrupted focus. It's a playful yet effective way to visualize and achieve digital restraint. Meanwhile, Focus@Will uses music scientifically designed to boost concentration, helping tune out distractions in office environments or at home.

Something uniquely valuable about these apps is their ability to personalize experiences. For example, some apps let users select background sounds, set reminders during high-stress times, or even participate in community challenges. This personalization fosters a sense of ownership and commitment to the process, making it more likely that users will stick with their new practices. By tailoring your practice to fit personal preferences, you're more inclined to incorporate mindfulness into your daily routine.

In the quest for balance, exploring a variety of mindfulness and focus apps can be enlightening. Simple Habit offers five-minute meditations for those who can't afford to sit still for long. Insight Timer boasts a vast library of guided sessions, music tracks, and talks by mindfulness experts worldwide. This diversity ensures that everyone can find a style and duration that suits their individual needs.

However, while these technologies offer great promise, mindful app usage is key. It's all too easy to become overwhelmed by the very tools meant to help. Therefore, strategically selecting the apps that align with your goals and resonate with your inner needs is vital. Just as with any tool, their effectiveness depends largely on how they are employed in service to your broader wellness journey.

There's also a communal aspect to many mindfulness apps that can't be overlooked. Features that connect users through shared goals or virtual meditation groups add depth to solitary practices. This virtual support network can motivate users and provide a platform for sharing experiences and insights, fostering a community of like-minded individuals who encourage and uplift each other.

Ultimately, utilizing these apps can transform how we relate to technology. They remind us that technology doesn't have to be the enemy of our mental well-being. Instead, it can become an ally in the pursuit of a more mindful, focused, and fulfilling life. By incorporating these tools thoughtfully, we can reshape our digital experiences to better serve our mental and emotional health.

As we embrace these innovations, we pave the way for a future where technology complements, rather than dominates, our lives. The goal is to strike a balance—a harmonious relationship where technology supports our quest to live with intention and presence. By integrating apps designed for mindfulness and focus, we take a significant step toward a more centered existence, enhancing not just our personal well-being but also the quality of our interactions with the world around us.

Tools for Enhancing Productivity

Imagine a world where technology works not as a relentless taskmaster but as a supportive ally. It's possible to transform our digital tools from sources of distraction into powerful catalysts of productivity. In a time when digital noise and infinite scrolling often drown out our focus, harnessing the right tools can make all the difference. While it might seem paradoxical, technology—when used judiciously—can be key to reducing stress and elevating personal productivity.

At the heart of leveraging technology for enhancing productivity lies a fundamental understanding: not all tools are beneficial, and more isn't always better. It's easy to get caught up in downloading the latest apps, hoping one will magically streamline work or personal life. Yet, the truth often lies in simplifying, not complicating. Going back to basics with technology that truly serves our needs—rather than enslaving us to continuous updates and notifications—paves the way for a more mindful approach.

Start by assessing your current toolkit. Are there applications you rarely use that only add clutter? Decluttering your digital landscape can provide almost immediate mental relief. When you've only got the essentials, your workflow becomes smoother, and distractions dwindle. This act of digital minimalism isn't about limiting potential but about focusing on possibilities that lead to a balanced digital life.

Next, prioritize tools that encourage deep work and focus, such as time-tracking apps or distraction blockers. These applications help guard against the pull of social media and other habitual interruptions. For instance, apps like Freedom or Focus@Will create an environment conducive to concentration by limiting access to distracting sites or providing background music designed for focus. The result? A clearer mind and an open path for your most essential tasks.

Collaboration tools should enhance, not hinder, team productivity. In the workplace, tools such as Slack and Trello streamline communication and project management, allowing teams to work synchronously without endless email threads. However, making these platforms work for you involves setting boundaries. Specify times when you'll be available to engage on these platforms and when you need to focus on deep work. Communicate these boundaries to your colleagues to foster mutual respect for focused time.

Additionally, consider automation tools that alleviate repetitive tasks. Applications like IFTTT (If This Then That) or Zapier can automate mundane tasks by linking different apps and services, freeing up mental energy for more critical work. Whether it's sorting emails, organizing files, or sending automated reminders, these tools can be configured to streamline daily operations without requiring constant attention.

Aside from task-oriented tools, those that promote wellbeing and mental clarity are equally vital for maintaining productivity. Meditation and mindfulness apps, such as Calm or Headspace, can be integrated into daily routines to help manage stress and refocus energy. Regular use of these apps can build resilience and improve the overall approach to work—shift from busyness to meaningful engagement.

While goal-setting is crucial, maintaining flexibility in how you achieve those goals is equally important. Tools that offer customizable frameworks, like Todoist or Notion, allow users to tailor their planning processes, adapting them to shifting priorities. This adaptability ensures that you're not locked into any single way of working but are instead empowered to evolve your approach as needs change.

The technology itself isn't inherently good or bad; it's how we use it that determines its impact on our productivity. By intentionally selecting and employing tools that align with our goals and values, we cultivate an environment where technology aids rather than obstructs. This mindful integration of technology into our lives leads to reduced mental strain and an enhanced sense of accomplishment.

As we continue to navigate through the digital age, integrating tools that enhance productivity becomes not just a skill but an art. It involves a blend of self-awareness, discipline, and a keen eye for practicality. When these elements come together, they set the stage for a harmonious relationship with technology, where we drive our work forward with clarity and intention rather than being swept away by the digital tide.

Chapter 24:
Redefining Success Beyond the Screen

In the quest to redefine success beyond the screen, we lean towards a world where slowness, simplicity, and fulfillment aren't measured by digital validation. It's about shifting our focus from the incessant hustle of online approval to moments of genuine joy and contentment. Imagine finding success in the whisper of the wind, the laughter during a meal shared, or an evening spent with a good book. In this chapter, we explore how embracing these seemingly small experiences can ground us, offering a counterbalance to the urgency of digital life. Letting go of the need for constant connection online opens us to a richer tapestry of living—a life in which success isn't a metric but a state of being present and at peace with ourselves. So, let's take a purposeful step back, prioritizing what truly matters and redefining what success means in this digital age.

Embracing Slowness and Simplicity

In this age of relentless digital acceleration, slowing down feels almost countercultural. Yet, it's through embracing a slower pace that we can truly redefine success beyond the screen. Imagine waking up without the immediate reach for your smartphone, savoring the quiet moments of the morning without data, notifications, or digital assumptions pulling at your attention. There is a profound richness in simplicity—a clarity that emerges only when distractions step aside.

Slowness and simplicity are not about abandoning all technology or resisting progress. Rather, they are about making conscious choices that align with our values. This involves taking moments to pause, reflecting on our relationship with technology, and asking ourselves: Are our digital habits serving our broader life goals, or are they dictating an unexamined path?

Consider how simplicity can transform productivity. When we're constantly jumping from one task to another, with screens perpetually blinking and buzzing, our cognitive resources spread thin. Embracing slowness allows us to concentrate on one task at a time, fostering deeper engagement and satisfaction. The power of this deliberate focus can't be overstated—it's the key to unlocking creativity and achieving meaningful outcomes.

The journey towards simplicity doesn't demand drastic lifestyle changes overnight. Instead, it's about small, intentional actions. Start by identifying the noise in your digital life. Which apps or tools genuinely contribute to your well-being? Which ones do you hold onto out of habit rather than necessity? By pruning digital clutter, you're clearing the mental space needed to appreciate and focus on what truly matters.

Every day, we encounter countless decisions that steer us either towards or away from wholeness. Embracing simplicity is about recognizing these choices, visible and invisible, and choosing pathways that cultivate peace. It involves a shift in our mindset—from one that values immediacy and efficiency to one that nurtures presence and mindfulness. This isn't a rejection of technology, but an affirmation of our capacity to live and thrive beyond its confines.

Simplicity thrives in the gaps of silence—those rare, treasured moments where you can hear your own thoughts. These spaces are where creativity grows and where the nuances of life become vibrant again. It's here that you can reconnect with passions and experiences that bring genuine joy. Without the rush, we find room to rediscover the beauty in everyday life, in conversations unburdened by digital intrusions, in nature walks unhurried by the thought of the next email or message.

There is something profoundly empowering in reclaiming time for ourselves. As we slow down, the tyranny of urgency diminishes. There's freedom in knowing that not every ping requires an immediate response and that not every update deserves our attention. We begin to trust in a slower, more deliberate rhythm—where the quality of experiences outweighs their quantity.

Embracing slowness also nurtures our mental health, acting as a balm against the backdrop of a world that often feels overwhelming. It offers a pathway to intersperse our days with moments of reflection and rest, encouraging a more sustainable pace that protects against burnout. By reconnecting with these slower rhythms, we foster resilience and a sense of abundance rather than scarcity.

We must acknowledge that simplicity is not synonymous with deprivation. Instead, it is an abundant way to engage with the world— one where each interaction holds purpose and meaning. Success, then, transcends conventional metrics defined by digital validation and returns to a more intrinsic sense of fulfillment. It is shaped by personal growth, authentic relationships, and a deep appreciation for the world around us.

Ultimately, the call to embrace slowness and simplicity is a call to live intentionally. It's about weaving moments into our lives where we can breathe, reflect, and simply be. It invites us to rewrite the narratives of busyness that often define our worth. As we do so, we uncover a landscape where life unfolds joyfully and powerfully beyond the confines of pixels and screens.

In this journey towards a slower, simpler life, may we remember that we're not alone. There is a growing community of individuals who, like us, are choosing to redefine success in more personal and profound ways. Let's connect, share, and support each other as we step boldly into a life where technology serves our deepest values rather than distracts from them.

Finding Fulfillment Outside of Digital Validation

In an era where "likes" and comments can drive our self-worth, it is essential to step back and reassess what truly constitutes fulfillment. We've grown accustomed to seeking validation through digital interaction, an environment engineered to keep us engaged and craving more. But the real richness of life often lies outside the confines of screens and digital acknowledgments.

Finding fulfillment beyond digital validation requires intentionality. It starts with identifying the aspects of life that don't rely on someone fitting our existence into the endless scroll of social media. This could mean pursuing hobbies that have no digital footprint or enjoying experiences that can't be quantified in metrics such as views or followers. For many, this involves reconnecting with passions that existed before technology became all-pervasive.

The allure of digital validation is rooted in its immediacy—it offers instant gratification and is ever-accessible. However, the depth and satisfaction we obtain from it are often fleeting. One way to counter this is by engaging in activities that require a more profound investment of time and effort, like cultivating a new skill or resuming former hobbies. Such pursuits often offer sustained joy and a sense of accomplishment that outlast a temporary digital thumbs-up.

Furthermore, the journey to fulfillment is not a solo race but a shared experience. Building authentic, face-to-face connections fortifies our lives in ways no digital interaction can. These relationships demand vulnerability and trust—elements often glossed over in curated online personas. There's something undeniably grounding about conversations that involve eye contact and shared laughter rather than emojis and memes.

Moreover, nature can be an incredible teacher in the quest for deeper fulfillment. It reminds us of the sheer simplicity and beauty found beyond our devices. Spending time in green spaces, observing the rhythm of the natural world, offers a welcomed contrast to the fast-paced digital frenzy. Nature's lack of judgment and its constancy provide a reminder of life's intrinsic value, independent of any external approval.

It's also worth considering how we use our digital time. Rather than endlessly consuming content, we might focus on creating it, not for external validation, but as a means of self-expression and personal satisfaction. Projects like writing, painting, or composing music can offer a profound sense of fulfillment purely through the process of creation itself. Through such endeavors, we often find our worth is not reliant on external applause but on our relationship with our own creativity.

Philosophical and spiritual teachings have long emphasized the importance of looking within rather than seeking outside approval. Mindfulness practices, meditation, and yoga are powerful ways to turn the focus inward. They help us understand that genuine contentment resides in the present moment and not in the endless pursuit of external accolades. Such practices help declutter the mental noise generated by digital devices, offering instead a silence that can be filled with self-reflection and realization.

At first, the absence of digital validation can feel like a void. The immediate feedback we're used to might create an initial sense of loss. However, with time, this space becomes fertile ground for growth. As the enticement of digital approval fades, the genuine enjoyment of life's little pleasures becomes more apparent. The small joys, like savoring a morning coffee without distraction or losing oneself in a book, carry a different weight when experienced fully and presently.

Redefining fulfillment is not about rejecting technology but about reprioritizing how we value and integrate it into our daily lives. By choosing to focus on experience over appearances, on lasting values over fleeting trends, we serve both ourselves and our broader community. This shift not only enhances personal well-being but also contributes to a more empathetic and grounded society.

To navigate this transition, one might set tangible goals, such as dedicating certain hours of the day to being entirely offline. Setting aside time for analogue activities or interactions can create a buffer from the constant lure of screens. By doing so, you'll find more space for introspection and genuine connections that don't require a Wi-Fi signal.

In the end, finding fulfillment outside of digital validation is about crafting a life that feels as good on the inside as it looks on the outside. It's about finding joy in the process rather than the product, valuing the journey as much as the destination. As challenging as it might seem, stepping off the digital carousel allows us to rediscover and redefine what success and happiness mean on our terms. And that might just be the most satisfying validation of all.

Chapter 25:
Sustainable Tech Habits for the Future

We've arrived at a pivotal moment where the choices we make about technology today will shape our collective tomorrow. By nurturing sustainable tech habits, we can carve out a future where the digital world seamlessly complements our physical lives, rather than overshadowing them. This means embracing practices that not only prioritize efficiency but also enrich our wellbeing. It's about developing long-term digital autonomy, enabling us to use technology as a tool, not a tether. As we foster a culture of mindfulness, we encourage intentional, purposeful interactions with our screens, creating room for creativity and presence that can't be measured by algorithms. Let's envision a future where our tech habits align with our deepest values, ensuring that the digital age serves humanity rather than the other way around. Together, we can build a world where technology enhances the human experience, paving the way for more meaningful connections and a balanced life.

Developing Long-term Digital Autonomy

In a world teeming with digital stimuli, the quest for long-term digital autonomy begins with understanding and redefining our relationship with technology. We all face the challenge of finding balance in a hyper-connected environment that constantly clamors for our attention. Yet, this balance is crucial for achieving a state of mind where technology serves as a tool, not a tyrant. By cultivating habits that promote digital autonomy, we can reclaim control over our digital experiences and foster a sense of well-being. This journey is not about cutting ties with technology but transforming the way we interact with it.

Digital autonomy is achieved by setting intentional usage habits that align with our personal values and life goals. It involves recognizing how technology fits into the broader tapestry of our lives, rather than letting it weave its own narrative. Embracing autonomy means making conscious choices about when and how to engage with digital devices, as well as recognizing when it's beneficial to unplug. This self-awareness is the cornerstone of living harmoniously with technology, nurturing an empowering connection that enhances our lives.

To develop long-term digital autonomy, it's imperative to start with small, actionable changes. This process might begin with scheduling daily tech-free time, enabling us to reconnect with our immediate environment and ourselves. Gradually, these increments of digital downtime can expand as you notice the benefits. It's about creating intentional pauses that allow our minds to reset and our creativity to flourish. Establishing these moments gives us the time to reflect and assess whether our digital habits align with what we truly value.

One of the most effective strategies for cultivating autonomy is embedding mindfulness into your digital interactions. Mindfulness encourages presence and deliberate action, preventing us from slipping into mindless scrolling or digital distractions. For example, before opening an app or checking an email, take a moment to breathe and consider why you're doing it. Question whether it serves your current objective or merely fills an idle moment. This practice roots you firmly in the present, promoting clarity rather than chaos.

Structured digital interventions—such as apps that track screen time, restrict certain features, or promote focused use—can aid in reinforcing these mindful habits. These tools help visualize your digital behavior patterns, providing insights into areas where change might be needed. They act as gentle reminders of your goals of autonomy, serving as virtual accountability partners. However, these should complement, not replace, the intrinsic discipline and awareness required for autonomy.

An often-overlooked aspect of developing digital autonomy is cultivating a supportive environment. Surround yourself with individuals who share your aspirations for healthier tech relationships. This community can offer mutual support, exchanging tips and celebrating progress. By fostering these connections, you create a culture that values intentionality and self-control in a digitally overwhelming world.

Revisiting your digital lifestyle regularly is another key to long-term autonomy. As your life and priorities evolve, so should your tech habits. What worked months ago may no longer serve your best interests. Periodic reflections on your goals ensure that your digital interactions remain aligned with your current needs. This flexibility not only strengthens your autonomy but also maintains an adaptive approach to technology that prevents stagnation.

Establishing boundaries is crucial in maintaining autonomy. Define spaces and times in your life where technology is off-limits, ensuring you are fully present in those moments. Whether it's during meals, family gatherings, or personal downtime, these boundaries safeguard your mental space from digital encroachment. They help reinforce the idea that while technology holds a place in our lives, it does not own all of it.

Long-term autonomy also hinges on educating ourselves about how technology shapes our behaviors and mindsets. Understanding the psychological mechanisms behind app design and social media can empower us to make better choices. Knowledge about these influences paves the way for skepticism and discernment, which are essential components of autonomy. With awareness comes the strength to choose wisely, ensuring technology complements rather than dictates our lives.

As we strive for autonomy, it's vital to remember that perfection isn't the goal. The process involves trial and error, celebrating small victories and learning from setbacks. It's about cultivating resilience to tech overwhelm, which allows you to bounce back and recalibrate when digital temptations arise. Approach this journey with self-compassion, acknowledging that growth takes time and patience.

Cultivating long-term digital autonomy ultimately leads to a more enriching and balanced life. It opens up space for creativity, genuine connections, and personal growth. Unshackled from the compulsions of digital dependency, we find more room to explore passions, engage with the world, and nurture meaningful relationships. By reclaiming control over our tech use, we transform our digital interactions into deliberate choices that foster a lasting sense of peace and fulfillment.

In this journey, technology becomes an enabler, not a detractor. It integrates seamlessly into our lives, supporting rather than distracting us from what truly counts. By taking deliberate steps towards digital autonomy, we pave the way for a future where technology serves as an ally in our quest for meaning and balance. This harmonious relationship with technology is not only sustainable but essential for a fulfilling life in the digital age.

Fostering a Culture of Mindfulness

In our digitally charged world, fostering a culture of mindfulness is not just a personal journey—it's a collective endeavor that promises a more sustainable relationship with technology. Mindfulness, at its core, is about being present. It's about developing an awareness of our thoughts, emotions, and physical surroundings without judgment. When applied to tech use, mindfulness encourages us to be intentional, to pause and reflect before we engage with our devices. This shift from mindless consumption to mindful engagement can transform our digital experiences and dramatically improve our overall well-being.

Mindfulness invites us to examine our motivations behind every tap, click, or swipe. Think about the last time you checked your phone. Did you do it because you received an important notification or simply out of habit? By recognizing the triggers that pull us into digital distraction, we can begin to question the necessity of our constant connectivity. This awareness is the first step toward creating healthier tech habits that align with our values rather than societal pressures.

A culture of mindfulness isn't cultivated in isolation. It starts with individual practices but must be supported by community norms and shared values. When communities prioritize time away from screens, they create environments where people feel empowered to disconnect without guilt. Families can foster mindfulness by establishing tech-free zones at home, colleagues by advocating for meeting-free blocks at work, and friends by choosing face-to-face interactions over digital communication. These small, collective actions contribute to a broader cultural shift where mindful tech use becomes the norm rather than the exception.

Transitioning toward this culture requires both commitment and patience. It's about expecting gradual progress rather than immediate transformation. Begin with simple steps like designating specific times of the day to unplug, practicing deep breathing exercises instead of reaching for your phone, or engaging in activities that ground you in the present moment, such as walking in nature or meditating. Over time, these practices fortify our ability to resist tech's allure and strengthen our commitment to living mindfully.

Introducing mindfulness into educational settings is particularly impactful. Schools and universities can play a vital role by integrating mindfulness training into their curricula, helping students develop digital literacy skills alongside traditional academic learning. Teaching young people to navigate technology with awareness not only enhances their focus but also fosters empathy and better decision-making skills. These lessons, learned early, can shape future generations who value the quality of their digital interactions as much as the quantity of their connections.

Though technology often feels at odds with mindfulness, there are many ways it can support mindful living. Whether through apps designed for meditation, or tools that track screen time, technology provides resources that can aid rather than detract from our quest for mindfulness. By consciously choosing how and when we use these tools, we leverage them to support our mindful intentions rather than letting them dominate our time and attention.

As we move towards a culture of mindfulness, it's also essential to recognize and advocate for structural changes. This includes urging tech companies to create more user-friendly interfaces that prioritize the user's mental health and well-being. Features like app usage reminders, customizable notification settings, and more transparent data policies empower users to take control of their tech experiences. As consumers, demanding these changes can push companies to design technology that supports mindful living.

The journey toward a mindful culture isn't just about reducing screen time. It's about fostering environments where technology enhances our lives rather than detracts from them. By nurturing a culture of mindfulness, we can transform our relationship with technology, leading to more intentional, balanced, and fulfilling lives.

As individuals and communities commit to mindfulness, we're not just changing how we interact with our devices; we're changing how we live in the digital age—more consciously, more purposefully, and with greater peace.

Conclusion

As we close this journey through the maze of our digital lives, it's essential to recognize that the aim isn't merely to escape the noise but to harmonize our existence with the evolving digital landscape. The path forward requires embracing an awareness that fosters both intentionality and compassion for ourselves and others. We've unraveled the complexities of digital distractions, explored the psychological impacts, and acknowledged the social forces at play. Now, it's about knitting these insights into the fabric of our daily routines, cultivating a balanced digital life that enhances our well-being.

The age of digital overload has brought about unprecedented challenges but also unique opportunities to redefine how we engage with technology. By recognizing the signs of digital fatigue and understanding the impact on our mental health, we lay the groundwork for a more conscious interaction with our devices. Letting go of the myth of multitasking, we reclaim our focus through mindfulness, reaping the benefits of a less cluttered digital existence.

We've ventured into the core principles of digital minimalism, unlocking the benefits that arise from a pared-down approach to tech use. Understanding how our devices hijack our attention demands that we respond with agency—by setting firm boundaries and creating spaces that prioritize core, meaningful connections. These intentional actions foster resilience, preventing the overwhelm that often accompanies unmanaged technology use.

166

Revisiting the journey, we delved into the art of digital decluttering and discovered how minimizing unnecessary digital load paves the way for greater clarity and purpose. Social media, once a noisy interloper, finds its place within the curated world of conscious engagement. Notifications, alerts, and interruptions transform from stressors to signals that work in our favor, custom-tailored to echo the rhythm of our lives.

Similarly, embracing offline alternatives and rekindling old passions reminds us of the joy and fulfillment found beyond screens, reviving the beauty of stillness and face-to-face interaction. Encouraging family and workplace digital detox policies further weaves together a fabric of connection and presence, cultivating environments that advocate for mental clarity and focus.

While technology is undeniably a double-edged sword, it can also be a tool for good when leveraged mindfully. We've seen how tech companies shape our digital experiences and how we can advocate for our digital well-being. By building communities of intentional tech users, we share successes and hold each other accountable in the pursuit of a balanced digital life.

Ultimately, this introspective journey invites us to redefine success beyond screens. Slowness, simplicity, and presence inspire a sense of fulfillment that digital validation often obscures. Embracing the now, nurturing intentional relationships, and fostering gratitude become our focal points as we cultivate long-term, sustainable habits for a future grounded in digital autonomy.

Our exploration has taught us that while technology will continue evolving, our relationship with it rests firmly within our control. By embracing the principles and practices we've discussed, we unlock the ability to not just survive but thrive in the digital age. Let's continue to navigate this intricate terrain with intention, courage, and optimism, boldly shaping a future where technology enriches our lives rather than dictates them.

Appendix A:
Resources for Further Reading

As you continue to explore a more mindful and balanced relationship with technology, you may find yourself seeking further insights and perspectives. Below is a curated list of resources that expand on the topics we've touched on, offering deeper dives into the realms of digital wellness, productivity, and minimalism. These books, articles, and online materials are designed to motivate, educate, and guide you on your journey toward digital mindfulness.

Books

"Digital Minimalism: Choosing a Focused Life in a Noisy World" by Cal Newport – This book delves into the philosophy of digital minimalism and offers practical advice on reducing digital clutter to enhance focus and well-being.

"The Shallows: What the Internet Is Doing to Our Brains" by Nicholas Carr – Carr explores the impact of the internet on cognition, providing a compelling narrative on how technology shapes our attention spans and mental processes.

"How to Break Up with Your Phone" by Catherine Price – A guide to creating a healthier relationship with your smartphone, packed with tips and a step-by-step plan for a phone detox.

Articles and Essays

"The New Tech Detox" by Rebecca Sultan – This article offers insights into the growing movement of tech detoxing and its benefits for mental health.

"Why We're Addicted to Technology" by Adam Alter – Examining the psychological reasons behind our tech dependencies, this essay provides an eye-opening look at modern technology's effects.

Online Resources

Center for Humane Technology – An organization offering a wealth of resources aimed at prompting a more ethical approach to technology design and usage.

Mindful Techies – A community promoting mindful use of technology through courses and events that encourage conscious digital engagement.

These resources, rich with ideas and knowledge, can further empower you to refine your digital habits. As you dive into these materials, remember, the ultimate goal is not to disconnect entirely but to foster a thoughtful, intentional engagement with technology.

www.ingramcontent.com/pod-product-compliance
Lightning Source LLC
Chambersburg PA
CBHW051241050326
40689CB00007B/1020